CHOOSING HEALTH HIGH SCHOOL

FITNESS AND HEALTH

chakra
essANA

Betty M. Hubbard, EdD, CHES

ETR Associates
Santa Cruz, California
1997

ETR Associates (Education, Training and Research) is a nonprofit organization committed to fostering the health, well-being and cultural diversity of individuals, families, schools and communities. The publishing program of ETR Associates provides books and materials that empower young people and adults with the skills to make positive health choices. We invite health professionals to learn more about our high-quality publishing, training and research programs by contacting us at P.O. Box 1830, Santa Cruz, CA 95061-1830, (800) 321-4407.

Betty M. Hubbard, EdD, CHES, is a professor of health sciences at the University of Central Arkansas in Conway. She holds a BSE in biology, an MS in counseling, an MSE in health education and has taught biology, science and health education in grades K through 12. She received a Presidential Citation from the Association for the Advancement of Health Education and served as a member of the Joint Committee for National Health Education Standards. In addition to university teaching responsibilities, she coordinates teacher training, conducts research and serves as an author and consultant for health education curricula and videos.

Choosing Health High School
    Abstinence
    Body Image and Eating Disorders
    Communication and Self-Esteem
    Fitness and Health
    STD and HIV
    Sexuality and Relationships
    Tobacco, Alcohol and Drugs
    Violence and Injury

Series Editor: Kathleen Middleton, MS, CHES
Text design: Graphic Elements
Illustrations: Ann Smiley

Printed in the United States of America

10 9 8 7 6 5 4 3
ISBN 1-56071-518-9

Title No. H680

CONTENTS

CONTENTS

CONTENTS

CONTENTS

CONTENTS

Masters

CONTENTS

ACKNOWLEDGMENTS

Choosing Health High School was made possible with the assistance of dedicated curriculum developers, teachers and health professionals. This program evolved from *Entering Adulthood*, the high school component of the *Contemporary Health Series*. The richness of this new program is demonstrated by the pool of talented professionals involved in both the original and the new versions.

Developers

Nancy Abbey
ETR Associates
Santa Cruz, California

Clint E. Bruess, EdD, CHES
University of Alabama at Birmingham
Birmingham, Alabama

Dale W. Evans, HSD, CHES
California State University, Long Beach
Long Beach, California

Susan C. Giarratano, EdD, CHES
California State University, Long Beach
Long Beach, California

Betty M. Hubbard, EdD, CHES
University of Central Arkansas
Conway, Arkansas

Lisa K. Hunter, PhD
Health & Education Communication Consultants
Berkeley, California

Susan J. Laing, MS, CHES
Department of Veterans Affairs Medical Center
Birmingham, Alabama

Donna Lloyd-Kolkin, PhD
Health & Education Communication Consultants
New Hope, Pennsylvania

Jeanie M. White, EdM, CHES
Education Consultant
Keizer, Oregon

Reviewers and Consultants

Brian Adams
Family Planning Council of Western Massachusetts
Northampton, Massachusetts

Janel Siebern Bartlett, MS, CHES
Dutchess County BOCES
Poughkeepsie, NY

Lori J. Bechtel, PhD
Pennsylvania State University, Altoona Campus
Altoona, Pennsylvania

Judith M. Boswell, RN, MS, CHES
University of New Mexico
Albuquerque, New Mexico

Marika Botha, PhD
Lewis and Clark State College
Lewiston, Idaho

Wanda Bunting
Newark Unified School District
Newark, California

John Daniels
Golden Sierra High School
Garden Valley, California

Joyce V. Fetro, PhD, CHES
San Francisco Unified School District
San Francisco, California

Mark L. Giese, EdD, FACSM
Northeastern State University
Tahlequah, Oklahoma

Karen Hart, MS, CHES
San Francisco Unified School District
San Francisco, California

Janet L. Henke
Old Court Middle School
Randallstown, Maryland

Russell G. Henke, MEd
Montgomery County Public Schools
Rockville, Maryland

Jon W. Hisgen, MS
Pewaukee Public Schools
Waukesha, Wisconsin

Bob Kampa
Gilroy High School
Gilroy, California

Freya Klein Kaufmann, MS, CHES
New York Academy of Medicine
New York, New York

David M. Macrina, PhD
University of Alabama at Birmingham
Birmingham, Alabama

Linda D. McDaniel, MS
Van Buren Middle School
Van Buren, Arkansas

Robert McDermott, PhD
University of South Florida
Tampa, Florida

ACKNOWLEDGMENTS

Carole McPherson, MA
Mentor Teacher Mission Hill Junior High School
Santa Cruz, California

Robert Mischell, MD
University of California, Berkeley
Berkeley, California

Donna Muto, MS
Mount Ararat School
Topsham, Maine

Priscilla Naworski, MS, CHES
California Department of Education
Healthy Kids Resource Center
Alameda County Office of Education
Alameda, California

Norma Riccobuono
La Paloma High School
Brentwood, California

Mary Rose-Colley, DEd, CHES
Lock Haven University
Lock Haven, Pennsylvania

Judith K. Scheer, MEd, EdS, CHES
Contra Costa County Office of Education
Walnut Creek, California

Michael A. Smith, MS, CHES
Long Beach Unified School District
Long Beach, California

Janet L. Sola, PhD
YWCA of the U.S.A.
New York, New York

Susan K. Telljohnn, HSD
University of Toledo
Toledo, Ohio

Donna J. Underwood, MS
Consulting Public Health Administrator
Champaign, Illinois

Peggy Woosley
Stuttgart Public Schools
Stuttgart, Arkansas

Dale Zevin, MA
Educational Consultant
Watsonville, California

PROGRAM OVERVIEW

COMPONENTS

> ### PROGRAM GOAL
> **Students will acquire the necessary skills and information to make healthy choices.**

Choosing Health High School consists of 8 Teacher/Student Resource books in critical topics appropriate for the high school health curriculum. *Think, Choose, Act Healthy, High School* provides creative activities to augment the basic program. There are also 13 *Health Facts* books that provide additional content information for teachers.

- **Teacher/Student Resource Books**—These 8 books address key health topics, content and issues for high school students. All teacher/student information, instructional process, assessment tools and student activity masters for the particular topic are included in each book.

- *Think, Choose, Act Healthy, High School*—This book provides 150 reproducible student activities that work hand in hand with the teacher/student resource books. They will challenge students to think and make their own personal health choices.

- *Health Facts* **Books**—These reference books provide clear, concise background information to support the resource books.

PROGRAM OVERVIEW

Health Facts Books Correlation	
Resource Books	Health Facts Books
Abstinence	Abstinence Sexuality
Body Image and Eating Disorders	Nutrition and Body Image
Communication and Self-Esteem	Self-Esteem and Mental Health
Fitness and Health	Fitness
STD and HIV	STD HIV Disease
Sexuality and Relationships	Sexuality
Tobacco, Alcohol and Drugs	Drugs Tobacco
Violence and Injury	Violence Injury Prevention

TEACHING STRATEGIES

Each resource book is designed so you can easily find the instructional content, process and skills. You can spend more time on teaching and less on planning. Special tools are provided to help you challenge your students, reach out to their families and assess student success.

A wide variety of learning opportunities is provided in each book to increase interest and meet the needs of different kinds of learners. Many are interactive, encouraging students to help each other learn. The **31** teaching strategies can be divided into 4 categories based on educational purpose. They are Informational, Creative Expression, Sharing Ideas and Opinions and Developing Critical Thinking. Descriptions of the teaching strategies are found in the appendix.

Providing Key Information

Students need information before they can move to higher-level thinking. This program uses a variety of strategies to provide the information students need to take actions for health. Strategies include:

- anonymous question box
- current events
- demonstrations
- experiments
- games and puzzles
- guest speakers
- information gathering
- interviewing
- oral presentations

Encouraging Creative Expression

Creative expression provides the opportunity to integrate language arts, fine arts and personal experience into learning. It also allows students the opportunity to demonstrate their understanding in ways that are unique to them. Creative expression encourages students to capitalize on their strengths and their interests. Strategies include:

- artistic expression
- creative writing
- dramatic presentations
- roleplays

TEACHING STRATEGIES

Sharing Ideas, Feelings and Opinions

In the sensitive area of health education, providing a safe atmosphere in which to discuss a variety of opinions and feelings is essential. Discussion provides the opportunity to clarify misinformation and correct misconceptions. Strategies include:

- brainstorming
- class discussion
- clustering
- continuum voting
- dyad discussion
- family discussion
- forced field analysis
- journal writing
- panel discussion
- self-assessment
- small groups
- surveys and inventories

Developing Critical Thinking

Critical thinking skills are crucial if students are to adopt healthy behaviors. Healthy choices necessitate the ability to become independent thinkers, analyze problems and devise solutions in real-life situations. Strategies include:

- case studies
- cooperative learning groups
- debates
- factual writing
- media analysis
- personal contracts
- research

PROGRAM OVERVIEW

SKILLS INFUSION

Studies of high-risk children and adolescents show that certain characteristics are common to children who succeed in adverse situations. These children are called resilient. Evaluation of educational programs designed to build resiliency has shown that several elements are important for success. The most important is the inclusion of activities designed to build personal and social skills.

Throughout each resource book, students practice skills along with the content addressed in the activities. Activities that naturally infuse personal and social skills are identified.

- **Communication**—Students with effective communication skills are able to express thoughts and feelings, actively listen to others, and give clear verbal and nonverbal messages related to health or any other aspect of their lives.

- **Decision Making**—Students with effective decision-making skills are able to identify decision points, gather information, and analyze and evaluate alternatives before they take action. This skill is important to promote positive health choices.

- **Assertiveness**—Students with effective assertiveness skills are able to resist pressure and influence from peers, advertising or others that may be in conflict with healthy behavior. This skill involves the ability to negotiate in stressful situations and refuse unwanted influences.

- **Stress Management**—Students with effective stress-management skills are able to cope with stress as a normal part of life. They are able to identify situations and conditions that produce stress and adopt healthy coping behaviors.

- **Goal Setting**—Students with effective goal-setting skills are able to clarify goals based on their needs and interests. They are able to set realistic goals, identify the sub-steps to goals, take action and evaluate their progress. They are able to learn from mistakes and change goals as needed.

WORKING WITH FAMILIES AND COMMUNITIES

A few general principles can help you be most effective in teaching about health:

- Establish a rapport with your students, their families and your community.
- Prepare yourself so that you are comfortable with the content and instructional process required to teach about fitness and health successfully.
- Be aware of state laws and guidelines established by your school district that relate to health.
- Invite parents and other family members to attend a preview of the materials.

Family involvement improves student learning. Encourage family members and other volunteers to help you in the classroom as you teach these activities.

THE FITNESS AND HEALTH RESOURCE BOOK

WHY TEACH ABOUT FITNESS?

Every day we make choices about physical activities that affect our level of fitness. Physical activity, in turn, has an impact on a wide range of physical, mental and social factors. The relationship of fitness to overall health is important; research has linked fitness to a wide variety of health-related conditions. Self-concept, stress, obesity, cardiovascular disease, diabetes and mental attitude are all influenced by physical activity. Physical activity plays a key role in preventing disease and promoting health.

The activities in this book are intended to assist students in enhancing their present and future levels of fitness. The instruction reflects the latest theories about assessment and enhancement of the components of fitness.

Fitness and High School Students

Research suggests that fitness levels of American youth have declined in recent years due to a change in lifestyle that reflects lower levels of activity. Because lifestyle behaviors are learned, teens need the opportunity to practice skills that help them achieve increased levels of fitness. Incorporating exercise into their lifestyles as teenagers enables youth to develop fitness skills that will help them maintain fitness throughout their lives.

These units provide an opportunity to coordinate health education with physical education classes to meet the objectives. Teachers may want to conduct some of the activities using a gymnasium or playing field, while other activities lend themselves to classroom instruction.

Remember to approach fitness activities with sensitivity to students' backgrounds, experiences and vulnerability to group expectations and pressures. Many students will be self-conscious about their level of fitness and/or their personal appearance. It is particularly important to provide students with privacy when conducting fitness assessments. Emphasize that assessments are not competitive. The goal of these activities is to help students improve individual fitness levels and gain an enjoyment of physical activity that will enhance health throughout their lives.

THE FITNESS AND HEALTH RESOURCE BOOK

WHY TEACH ABOUT FITNESS?

Background Information About Fitness

Instant Expert sections throughout this book give you all the information you need to teach each unit.

THE FITNESS AND HEALTH RESOURCE BOOK

OBJECTIVES

Students Will Be Able to:

Unit 1: The Meaning of Fitness
- List 3 benefits of fitness.
- Describe the elements of fitness.

Unit 2: Feeling Good About Myself
- Evaluate body image.
- Demonstrate behaviors that enhance the body image of others.

Unit 3: On Your Mark, Get Set, Go!
- Analyze their individual levels of fitness.

Unit 4: In a Heartbeat
- Synthesize a plan to improve aerobic capacity.

Unit 5: Looking Good—Feeling Good
- Analyze ways to improve body composition, flexibility, muscular strength and endurance.
- Analyze fitness facilities or programs in the community.

Unit 6: Be Prepared
- Identify common myths associated with fitness.
- Describe factors that influence the success of a fitness program.

Unit 7: Putting It All Together
- Identify personal goals for fitness.
- Develop a personal exercise plan.
- Evaluate the effectiveness of a personal fitness plan.

ANATOMY OF A UNIT

PREPARING TO TEACH

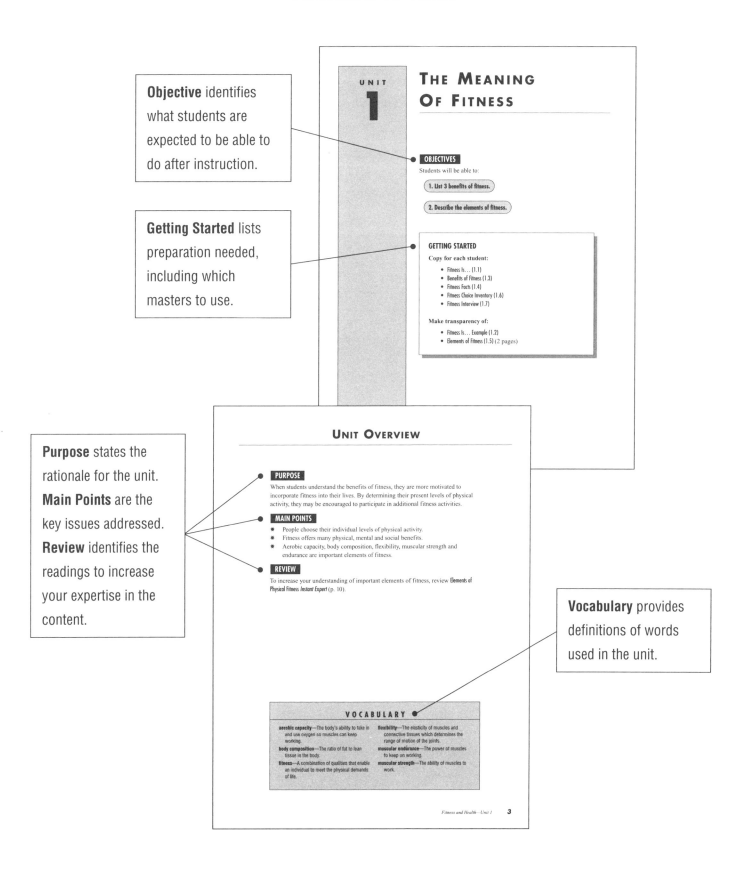

Objective identifies what students are expected to be able to do after instruction.

Getting Started lists preparation needed, including which masters to use.

Purpose states the rationale for the unit. **Main Points** are the key issues addressed. **Review** identifies the readings to increase your expertise in the content.

Vocabulary provides definitions of words used in the unit.

UNIT 1

THE MEANING OF FITNESS

OBJECTIVES
Students will be able to:

1. List 3 benefits of fitness.
2. Describe the elements of fitness.

GETTING STARTED
Copy for each student:
- Fitness Is… (1.1)
- Benefits of Fitness (1.3)
- Fitness Facts (1.4)
- Fitness Choice Inventory (1.6)
- Fitness Interview (1.7)

Make transparency of:
- Fitness Is… Example (1.2)
- Elements of Fitness (1.5) (2 pages)

UNIT OVERVIEW

PURPOSE
When students understand the benefits of fitness, they are more motivated to incorporate fitness into their lives. By determining their present levels of physical activity, they may be encouraged to participate in additional fitness activities.

MAIN POINTS
* People choose their individual levels of physical activity.
* Fitness offers many physical, mental and social benefits.
* Aerobic capacity, body composition, flexibility, muscular strength and endurance are important elements of fitness.

REVIEW
To increase your understanding of important elements of fitness, review Elements of Physical Fitness Instant Expert (p. 10).

VOCABULARY

aerobic capacity—The body's ability to take in and use oxygen so muscles can keep working.
body composition—The ratio of fat to lean tissue in the body.
fitness—A combination of qualities that enable an individual to meet the physical demands of life.

flexibility—The elasticity of muscles and connective tissues which determines the range of motion of the joints.
muscular endurance—The power of muscles to keep on working.
muscular strength—The ability of muscles to work.

Fitness and Health—Unit 1 **3**

ANATOMY OF A UNIT

TEACHING THE ACTIVITIES

Instant Expert pages provide concise background information for you. They follow each unit.

Process Cue identifies the teaching strategy used for the activity. Descriptions are in the Teaching Strategies appendix.

Building Skills icons identify activities that provide skill-specific practice.

Sharpen the Skill suggests ideas for more skills practice.

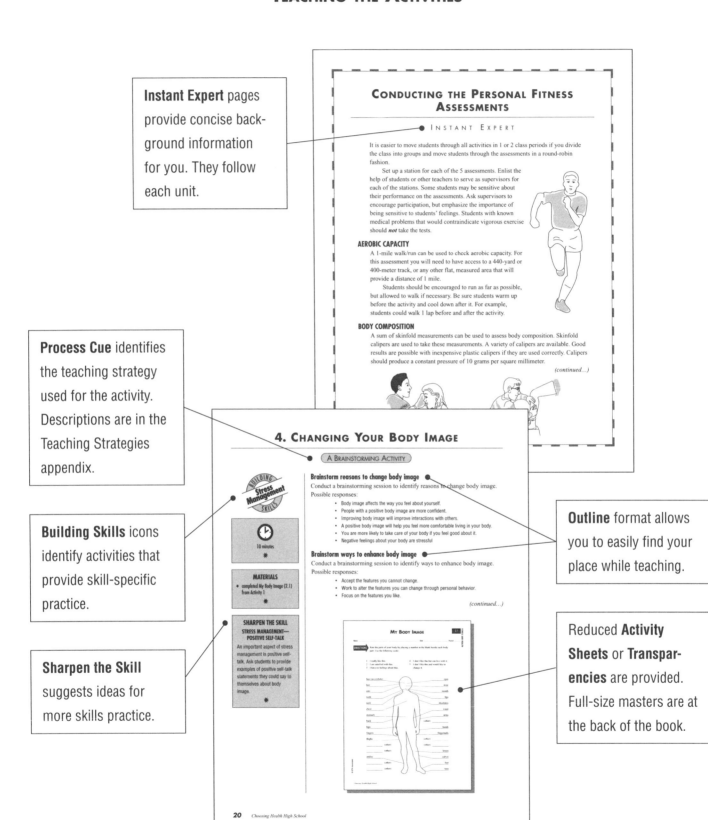

CONDUCTING THE PERSONAL FITNESS ASSESSMENTS

● INSTANT EXPERT

It is easier to move students through all activities in 1 or 2 class periods if you divide the class into groups and move students through the assessments in a round-robin fashion.

Set up a station for each of the 5 assessments. Enlist the help of students or other teachers to serve as supervisors for each of the stations. Some students may be sensitive about their performance on the assessments. Ask supervisors to encourage participation, but emphasize the importance of being sensitive to students' feelings. Students with known medical problems that would contraindicate vigorous exercise should *not* take the tests.

AEROBIC CAPACITY
A 1-mile walk/run can be used to check aerobic capacity. For this assessment you will need to have access to a 440-yard or 400-meter track, or any other flat, measured area that will provide a distance of 1 mile.

Students should be encouraged to run as far as possible, but allowed to walk if necessary. Be sure students warm up before the activity and cool down after it. For example, students could walk 1 lap before and after the activity.

BODY COMPOSITION
A sum of skinfold measurements can be used to assess body composition. Skinfold calipers are used to take these measurements. A variety of calipers are available. Good results are possible with inexpensive plastic calipers if they are used correctly. Calipers should produce a constant pressure of 10 grams per square millimeter.

(continued...)

4. CHANGING YOUR BODY IMAGE

(A BRAINSTORMING ACTIVITY)

Brainstorm reasons to change body image ●
Conduct a brainstorming session to identify reasons to change body image. Possible responses:
- Body image affects the way you feel about yourself.
- People with a positive body image are more confident.
- Improving body image will improve interactions with others.
- A positive body image will help you feel more comfortable living in your body.
- You are more likely to take care of your body if you feel good about it.
- Negative feelings about your body are stressful

Brainstorm ways to enhance body image ●
Conduct a brainstorming session to identify ways to enhance body image. Possible responses:
- Accept the features you cannot change.
- Work to alter the features you can change through personal behavior.
- Focus on the features you like.

(continued...)

🕐 **10 minutes**

MATERIALS
- completed My Body Image (2.1) from Activity 1

SHARPEN THE SKILL
STRESS MANAGEMENT—
POSITIVE SELF-TALK
An important aspect of stress management is positive self-talk. Ask students to provide examples of positive self-talk statements they could say to themselves about body image.

MY BODY IMAGE

20 *Choosing Health High School*

Outline format allows you to easily find your place while teaching.

Reduced **Activity Sheets** or **Transparencies** are provided. Full-size masters are at the back of the book.

ANATOMY OF A UNIT

SPECIAL FEATURES

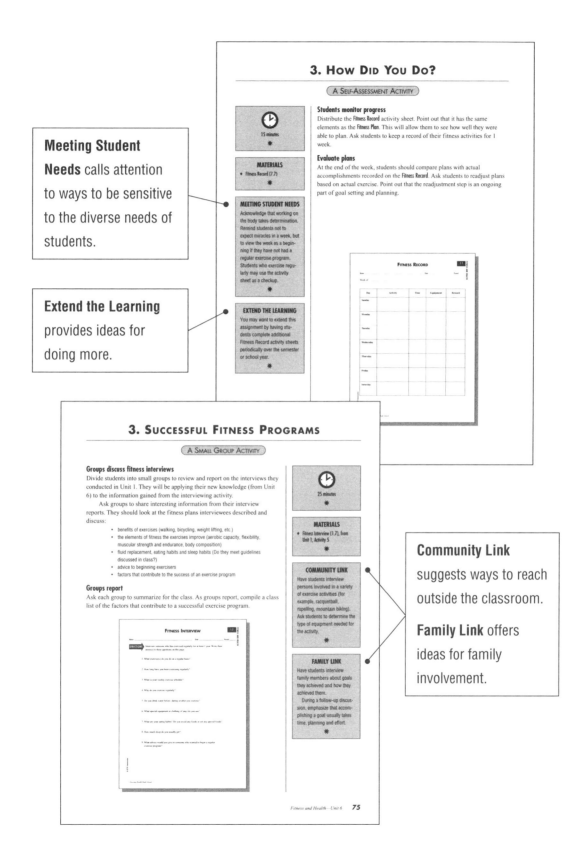

Meeting Student Needs calls attention to ways to be sensitive to the diverse needs of students.

Extend the Learning provides ideas for doing more.

3. HOW DID YOU DO?

A SELF-ASSESSMENT ACTIVITY

15 minutes

MATERIALS
♦ Fitness Record (7.7)

MEETING STUDENT NEEDS
Acknowledge that working on the body takes determination. Remind students not to expect miracles in a week, but to view the week as a beginning if they have not had a regular exercise program. Students who exercise regularly may use the activity sheet as a checkup.

EXTEND THE LEARNING
You may want to extend this assignment by having students complete additional Fitness Record activity sheets periodically over the semester or school year.

Students monitor progress
Distribute the Fitness Record activity sheet. Point out that it has the same elements as the Fitness Plan. This will allow them to see how well they were able to plan. Ask students to keep a record of their fitness activities for 1 week.

Evaluate plans
At the end of the week, students should compare plans with actual accomplishments recorded on the Fitness Record. Ask students to readjust plans based on actual exercise. Point out that the readjustment step is an ongoing part of goal setting and planning.

FITNESS RECORD

Day	Activity	Time	Equipment	Reward
Sunday				
Monday				
Tuesday				
Wednesday				
Thursday				
Friday				
Saturday				

3. SUCCESSFUL FITNESS PROGRAMS

A SMALL GROUP ACTIVITY

Groups discuss fitness interviews
Divide students into small groups to review and report on the interviews they conducted in Unit 1. They will be applying their new knowledge (from Unit 6) to the information gained from the interviewing activity.

Ask groups to share interesting information from their interview reports. They should look at the fitness plans interviewees described and discuss:

- benefits of exercises (walking, bicycling, weight lifting, etc.)
- the elements of fitness the exercises improve (aerobic capacity, flexibility, muscular strength and endurance, body composition)
- fluid replacement, eating habits and sleep habits (Do they meet guidelines discussed in class?)
- advice to beginning exercisers
- factors that contribute to the success of an exercise program

Groups report
Ask each group to summarize for the class. As groups report, compile a class list of the factors that contribute to a successful exercise program.

25 minutes

MATERIALS
♦ Fitness Interview (1.7), from Unit 1, Activity 5

COMMUNITY LINK
Have students interview persons involved in a variety of exercise activities (for example, racquetball, rapelling, mountain biking). Ask students to determine the type of equipment needed for the activity.

FAMILY LINK
Have students interview family members about goals they achieved and how they achieved them. During a follow-up discussion, emphasize that accomplishing a goal usually takes time, planning and effort.

Community Link suggests ways to reach outside the classroom.

Family Link offers ideas for family involvement.

FITNESS INTERVIEW

Fitness and Health—Unit 6 **75**

ANATOMY OF A UNIT

EVALUATION FEATURES

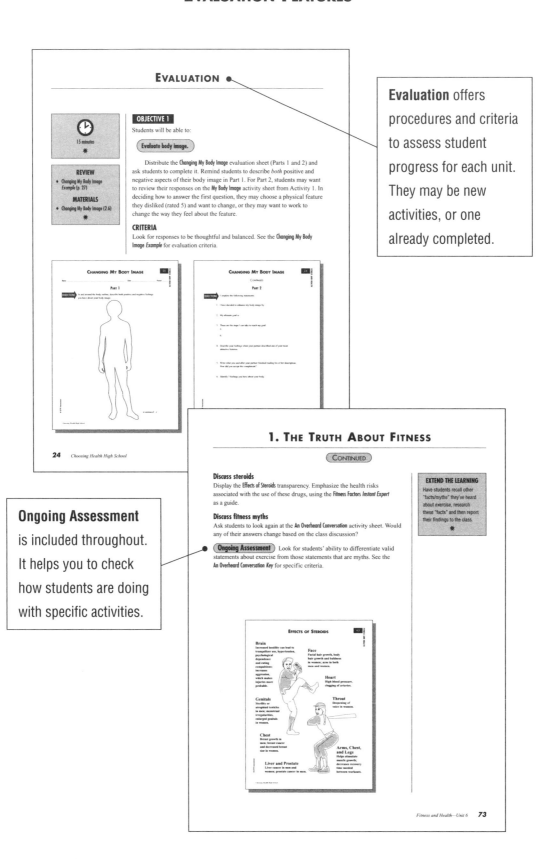

Evaluation offers procedures and criteria to assess student progress for each unit. They may be new activities, or one already completed.

Ongoing Assessment is included throughout. It helps you to check how students are doing with specific activities.

THE MEANING OF FITNESS

TIME

3 periods

ACTIVITIES

1. What Is Fitness?
2. The Elements of Fitness
3. Making Choices
4. Why Do You Exercise?

THE MEANING OF FITNESS

OBJECTIVES

Students will be able to:

1. List 3 benefits of fitness.

2. Describe the elements of fitness.

GETTING STARTED

Copy for each student:

- Fitness Is... (1.1)
- Benefits of Fitness (1.3)
- Fitness Facts (1.4)
- Fitness Choice Inventory (1.6)
- Fitness Interview (1.7)

Make transparency of:

- Fitness Is... Example (1.2)
- Elements of Fitness (1.5) (2 pages)

UNIT OVERVIEW

PURPOSE

When students understand the benefits of fitness, they are more motivated to incorporate fitness into their lives. By determining their present levels of physical activity, they may be encouraged to participate in additional fitness activities.

MAIN POINTS

✴ People choose their individual levels of physical activity.

✴ Fitness offers many physical, mental and social benefits.

✴ Aerobic capacity, body composition, flexibility, muscular strength and endurance are important elements of fitness.

REVIEW

To increase your understanding of important elements of fitness, review **Elements of Physical Fitness** *Instant Expert* (p. 10).

VOCABULARY

aerobic capacity—The body's ability to take in and use oxygen so muscles can keep working.

body composition—The ratio of fat to lean tissue in the body.

fitness—A combination of qualities that enable an individual to meet the physical demands of life.

flexibility—The elasticity of muscles and connective tissues which determines the range of motion of the joints.

muscular endurance—The power of muscles to keep on working.

muscular strength—The ability of muscles to work.

1. WHAT IS FITNESS?

25 minutes

MATERIALS

♦ Fitness Is… (1.1)
♦ transparency of Fitness Is… Example (1.2)
♦ Benefits of Fitness (1.3)

A BRAINSTORMING AND CLUSTERING ACTIVITY

Define fitness

Ask students what fitness means to them. Distribute the Fitness Is… activity sheet, and display the Fitness Is… *Example* transparency. Ask students to brainstorm words that come to mind when they think about fitness. Explain clustering, and allow students time to complete the activity sheet. (See the Teaching Strategies Appendix for a description of clustering.)

Discuss fitness benefits

When students have completed their clusters, ask them if any of the terms they have written refer to the benefits of fitness (e.g., fun, healthy, feeling good, looking good). List student responses on a blank transparency or the board.

(continued…)

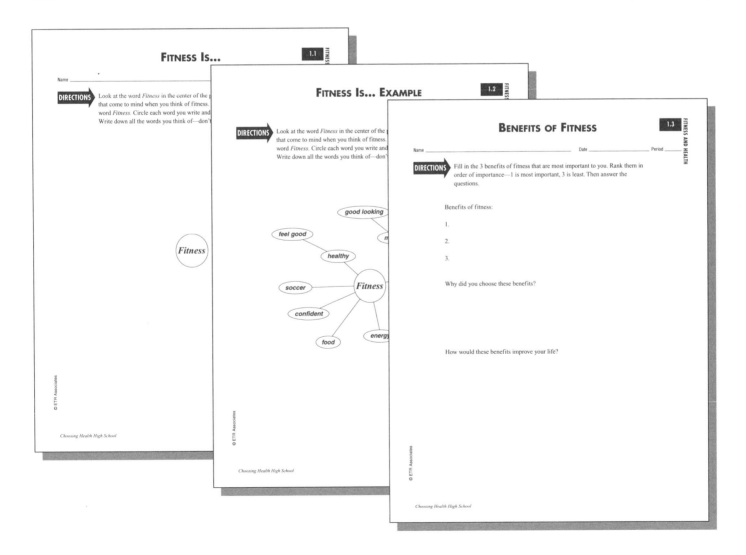

1. WHAT IS FITNESS?

CONTINUED

Ask students to add any additional benefits related to fitness. The completed list could include:

- stronger heart
- lower body fat
- stress reduction
- better sleep
- lower blood pressure
- higher self-esteem
- improved appearance
- more energy
- fewer diseases
- longer life

- lower cholesterol level
- improved digestion
- fewer injuries
- more positive outlook
- healthier immune system
- stronger bones
- improved muscle tone
- improved skin
- increased self-confidence
- improved mental ability

Students analyze benefits

Distribute the **Benefits of Fitness** activity sheet. Ask students to choose the 3 benefits of fitness that they would most like to include in their own lives. Have students fill in these benefits on the activity sheet and rank them from 1 to 3, with 1 being the most desirable.

Ask students to answer the questions that follow. When they have finished, ask for volunteers to share their responses with the class and to explain the basis of their rankings.

Ongoing Assessment Look for student responses to demonstrate a conceptual understanding that fitness promotes a positive self-image, helps protect against health problems, and generally enhances the ability to meet the demands of daily living.

EXTEND THE LEARNING

Have students watch television commercials, looking for those that use appearance or physical abilities to sell products. Students should employ critical-thinking skills to analyze and evaluate the commercials they watch. Brainstorm a list of questions to assist in analyzing the commercials. Examples:

- Does the product improve fitness?
- How did the advertisement try to persuade the viewer to buy the product?

Have students write about their experiences. Ask them to make a statement about the value of the commercial, using details from their analysis to support their evaluation.

2. THE ELEMENTS OF FITNESS

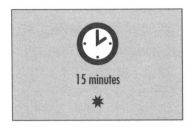

15 minutes

MATERIALS

◆ Fitness Facts (1.4)
◆ transparencies of Elements of Fitness (1.5)

Discuss elements of fitness

Distribute the Fitness Facts activity sheet, and display the Elements of Fitness transparencies. Discuss each element, using the Elements of Physical Fitness *Instant Expert* as a guide. Ask students to write on the activity sheet, in their own words, the definition of each element as you explain the meaning of the terms.

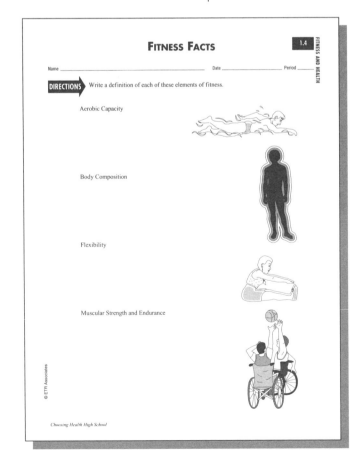

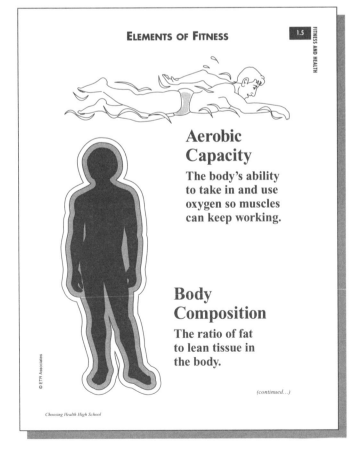

3. MAKING CHOICES

Students assess activity levels

Distribute the **Fitness Choice Inventory** activity sheet to help students evaluate their current level of physical activity. Ask students to answer the questions. Encourage them to answer the questions without looking at the scoring criteria. After they have made their choices on the questions, they should score their responses.

Discuss activity levels

Lead a class discussion about the choices people make regarding activity levels. Ask students:

- Was your score higher or lower than you expected?
- Are you pleased with your score?
- Are there some easy ways to get more physical activity in your life?
- What activities contribute the most physical activity to your daily life?

Ongoing Assessment Look for students' ability to identify strategies to incorporate fitness activities into their daily lives, such as walking to and from school, using stairs, etc.

15 minutes

MATERIALS

♦ Fitness Choice Inventory (1.6)

FAMILY LINK

Invite students to administer the Fitness Choice Inventory to family members. Without names, review the results of the inventories. Challenge students to draw conclusions about the results.

MEETING STUDENT NEEDS

Discourage sharing *any* specific information about student inventory scores. This information is personal and an environment of respect for privacy must be established. Student scores on the inventory will vary. Emphasize that any physical activity is beneficial.

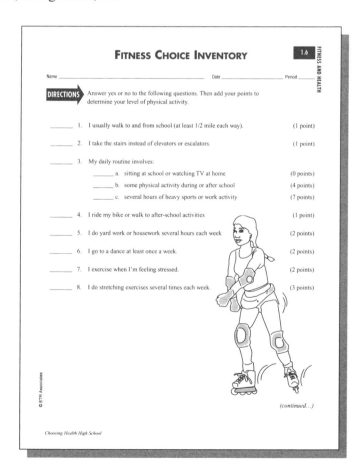

4. WHY DO YOU EXERCISE?

AN INTERVIEWING ACTIVITY

20 minutes

MATERIALS
◆ Fitness Interview (1.7)

EXTEND THE LEARNING

Assign students to shop for exercise equipment (for example, jogging shoes, ski equipment, hiking equipment). Ask them to determine price and other important information about the products (e.g., how many gears are necessary on a mountain bike? What type tires are preferred and why?)

Students interview exercisers

Distribute the Fitness Interview activity sheet. Ask students to interview an individual who has exercised regularly for at least 1 year. Encourage students to interview a variety of people, including people of different ages and genders and people who do different types of exercise.

Discuss interviews

Conduct a class discussion on the interviews. Ask students:
- What did you learn from the interview?
- Did anything surprise you?
- What conclusions can you draw based on these interviews?

Explain that although some people may choose fitness facilities as a way to improve or maintain their fitness, many people plan their fitness programs around activities that are always available and free.

Ongoing Assessment Look for students to recognize the uniqueness in personal preferences for fitness programs or activities. The key is the ability to match needs and wants to a personal fitness plan.

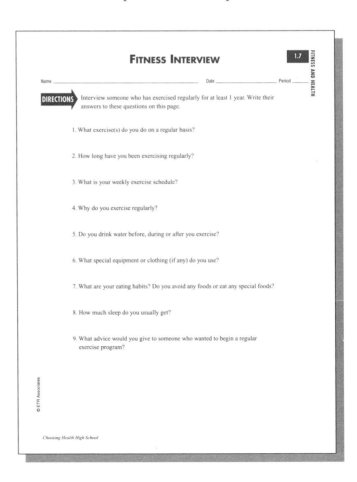

FITNESS INTERVIEW · 1.7

Name _____ Date _____ Period _____

DIRECTIONS Interview someone who has exercised regularly for at least 1 year. Write their answers to these questions on this page.

1. What exercise(s) do you do on a regular basis?

2. How long have you been exercising regularly?

3. What is your weekly exercise schedule?

4. Why do you exercise regularly?

5. Do you drink water before, during or after you exercise?

6. What special equipment or clothing (if any) do you use?

7. What are your eating habits? Do you avoid any foods or eat any special foods?

8. How much sleep do you usually get?

9. What advice would you give to someone who wanted to begin a regular exercise program?

© ETR Associates

Choosing Health High School

EVALUATION

OBJECTIVE 1

Students will be able to:

> **List 3 benefits of fitness.**

Assess students' responses on the **Benefits of Fitness** activity sheet for their ability to identify at least 3 benefits of fitness.

CRITERIA

See the **Elements of Physical Fitness** *Instant Expert* for assessment criteria. Responses may include:

- health
- stress management
- physical appearance
- "feeling good"
- energy
- fun

REVIEW

◆ Elements of Physical Fitness *Instant Expert* (p. 10)

MATERIALS

◆ completed Benefits of Fitness (1.3), from Activity 1

OBJECTIVE 2

Students will be able to:

> **Describe the elements of fitness.**

Assess student responses on the **Fitness Facts** activity sheet for their ability to describe each of the elements of fitness.

CRITERIA

See the **Elements of Physical Fitness** *Instant Expert* for evaluation criteria. Look for responses that use students' own words to define:

- aerobic capacity
- body composition
- flexibility
- muscular strength
- endurance

REVIEW

◆ Elements of Physical Fitness *Instant Expert* (p. 10)

MATERIALS

◆ completed Fitness Facts (1.4), from Activity 2

ELEMENTS OF PHYSICAL FITNESS

Physical fitness is one of the primary components of good health. Fitness enhances one's ability to meet the demands of daily living, cope with unexpected extra demands, have a realistic but positive self-image and protect oneself against health problems. Choices people make every day determine their level of fitness. Fitness continually changes in response to health behaviors such as diet and physical activity.

Aerobic capacity, body composition, flexibility, muscular strength and endurance are the main elements of physical fitness. Each of these elements can be enhanced by a regular exercise program.

AEROBIC CAPACITY

Aerobic capacity is the foundation for whole-body fitness. It is the body's ability to take in and use oxygen so that muscles can keep working. The level of aerobic capacity depends on the ability of the heart muscle and lungs to supply oxygen to the cells in the body, and the ability of the cells to efficiently use the oxygen and eliminate carbon dioxide.

Most experts agree that aerobic capacity is the most important element of fitness. Engaging in aerobic exercise on a regular basis is the best way to enhance aerobic capacity. By enhancing this element of fitness, a person improves the efficiency of the heart muscle and lungs, in addition to all of the other muscles in the body.

Currently, cardiovascular diseases (heart attack, stroke, atherosclerosis) are the leading cause of death for Americans. Research shows that individuals who engage in a regular exercise program that improves aerobic capacity can reduce their risk of developing these diseases. Starting an exercise program is especially important for young people. Scientists have discovered that cardiovascular diseases may begin during youth.

BODY COMPOSITION

Body composition refers to the ratio of body fat to lean tissue (muscle, bone, skin and internal organs). For good health, the body should have a proper ratio of one to the other. Body fat consists of 2 types: essential (brown) and storage (yellow). Essential fat is found in the vital organs, such as the lungs, heart, liver, spleen, kidneys and intestines. This fat protects these organs from injury and aids in important body processes. Storage fat accumulates around the internal organs, within muscle tissue and under the skin. Too much storage fat has been linked to cardiovascular disease, diabetes, cancer and arthritis.

(continued)

ELEMENTS OF PHYSICAL FITNESS

FLEXIBILITY

Flexibility is the ability of joints to move through their full range of motion. This movement at the joints enables a person to bend, touch the toes or rotate the body. Flexibility is influenced by gender (females are more flexible than males), age, posture and amount of fat and muscle. People become more flexible until adolescence, when the levels of flexibility begin to decline.

Flexibility depends on the elasticity of the connective tissues (tendons and ligaments) and muscles, and the condition of the joints. If flexibility is maintained, the body can move and bend instead of becoming injured in response to movements. In addition, the movements of flexible bodies are graceful and attractive. Flexibility can be improved through stretching.

MUSCULAR STRENGTH AND ENDURANCE

Muscular strength refers to the ability of the muscles to work—for example, to push a stalled car or to pick up a heavy load. Muscular endurance is the power of a muscle to keep on working. Muscular strength and endurance are necessary for everyday tasks, like mowing the yard or playing basketball.

Well-conditioned muscles work more smoothly and with less effort. The muscle tissue is firmer and can withstand more strain. Muscles never stay the same. If they are not used, they break down. With vigorous and regular exercise, they grow stronger.

FEELING GOOD ABOUT MYSELF

TIME

1–2 periods

ACTIVITIES

FEELING GOOD ABOUT MYSELF

OBJECTIVES

Students will be able to:

> 1. Evaluate body image.

> 2. Demonstrate behaviors that enhance the body image of others.

GETTING STARTED

Copy for each student:

- My Body Image (2.1)
- What Can't Be Changed *Case Studies* (2.2)
- Willing to Change *Case Studies* (2.3)
- Body Image Assessment (2.4)
- Partner Portrait (2.5)
- Changing My Body Image (2.6) (2 pages)

Copy:

- Roleplay Cards (2.7)

SPECIAL STEPS

Cut apart the **Roleplay Cards** and paste on 3" × 5" cards. See Evaluation (p. 25).

UNIT OVERVIEW

PURPOSE

This lesson serves as a preface for subsequent lessons that include assessments of physical fitness. Whenever physical assessments are conducted, some students will feel self-conscious about their bodies. In this lesson, students are reassured that feeling worried or uncomfortable about physical features is common, and are encouraged to be sensitive to others' feelings around body image.

MAIN POINTS

* Body image is the mental picture we have of our physical selves.
* Body image can be changed.
* We can influence the body image others have of themselves.

REVIEW

To increase your understanding of body image issues, review **Body Image** *Instant Expert* (p. 26) and **Changing My Body Image** *Example* (p. 27).

VOCABULARY

body image—The mental picture we have of our physical selves.

self-esteem—The way people feel about themselves.

1. WHAT'S YOUR PICTURE?

A SELF-ASSESSMENT ACTIVITY

15 minutes

MATERIALS

◆ My Body Image (2.1)

FAMILY LINK

Have students interview family members about physical features they like and dislike about themselves, including how their image of themselves has changed over the years. What conclusions can students draw from these interviews?

Discuss general conclusions in class. However, discourage sharing of specific or personal information. Ask students to make general statements.

Students rate physical features

Distribute the **My Body Image** activity sheet. Ask students to rate the parts of their bodies from 1 to 5, according to the scale provided. Emphasize that this is a *private* exercise to help them identify how they feel about their bodies. Activity sheet responses will *not* be shared.

Students differentiate features

Ask students to look at the physical features they rated 5 (features they dislike). Ask them to draw a box around those features they dislike that *cannot* be changed by their personal behavior (e.g., height, eye color, etc.).

Then have students draw a circle around features they dislike (those rated 5) that *can* be changed by personal behavior. For example, a person can tone muscles by exercising or use hair dye to change hair color.

Some discussion may center on changes that can be accomplished through surgery (e.g., breast augmentation and reduction, change in size and shape of nose, etc.). Try to keep the focus on changes students can make themselves through behavior.

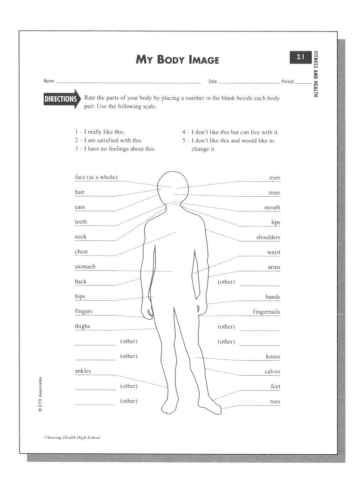

2. WHAT CAN BE CHANGED?

Discuss physical features that can't be changed

Explain that people have 2 choices regarding the physical features they dislike that cannot be changed. They can refuse to accept their bodies as they are and continue to feel bad about this (which can contribute to low self-esteem). *Or* they can change the way they think and feel about those particular physical features.

Groups discuss case studies

Divide the class into small groups. Distribute the **What Can't Be Changed** *Case Studies*. Explain the group assignment:

- Read the case studies.
- Discuss each case study and the questions that follow.

(continued...)

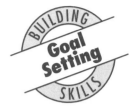

20 minutes

MATERIALS

- What Can't Be Changed *Case Studies* (2.2)
- Willing to Change *Case Studies* (2.3)

SHARPEN THE SKILL

GOAL SETTING— ACHIEVABLE GOALS

Conduct a discussion on the importance of identifying achievable goals. Ask students to reflect about this in relation to the case studies.

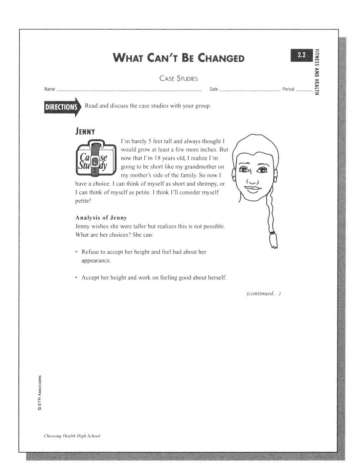

WHAT CAN'T BE CHANGED `2.2`

CASE STUDIES

Name _____ Date _____ Period _____

DIRECTIONS Read and discuss the case studies with your group.

JENNY

I'm barely 5 feet tall and always thought I would grow at least a few more inches. But now that I'm 18 years old, I realize I'm going to be short like my grandmother on my mother's side of the family. So now I have a choice. I can think of myself as short and shrimpy, or I can think of myself as petite. I think I'll consider myself petite!

Analysis of Jenny

Jenny wishes she were taller but realizes this is not possible. What are her choices? She can:

- Refuse to accept her height and feel bad about her appearance.

- Accept her height and work on feeling good about herself.

(continued...)

2. WHAT CAN BE CHANGED?

EXTEND THE LEARNING
Have students research ways in which different cultures attempt to enhance their physical attractiveness. For example, tattooing, body piercing, hairstyles and clothing.

Discuss changing features

Ask students to consider the physical features they circled on the **My Body Image** activity sheet—features they dislike that can be changed through personal behavior. Point out that students also have a choice about these features:

- They can keep the same behavior and continue to feel bad about these body parts.
- They can keep the same behavior and accept their appearance.
- They can change their behavior to help alter these features.

Groups discuss case studies

Distribute the **Willing to Change** *Case Studies*. Explain the group assignment:

- Read the case studies.
- Discuss each case study and the questions that follow.

Ongoing Assessment   Look for students' understanding that certain physical features, such as height, cannot be changed. They should also understand that it may be possible to change other physical features, such as muscle tone, by changing behavior.

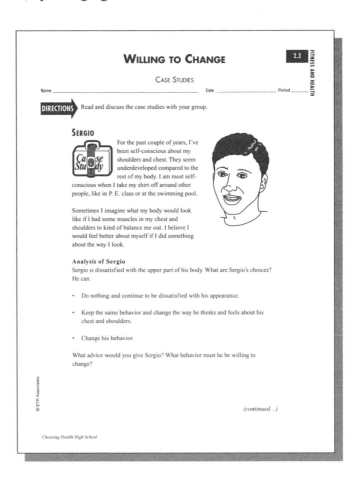

3. THINKING ABOUT BODY IMAGE

A SELF-ASSESSMENT ACTIVITY

Students summarize feelings

Distribute the **Body Image Assessment** activity sheet and ask students to complete it individually. Ask them to think about whether their responses are generally more positive or negative.

10 minutes

✳

MATERIALS

◆ Body Image Assessment (2.4)

✳

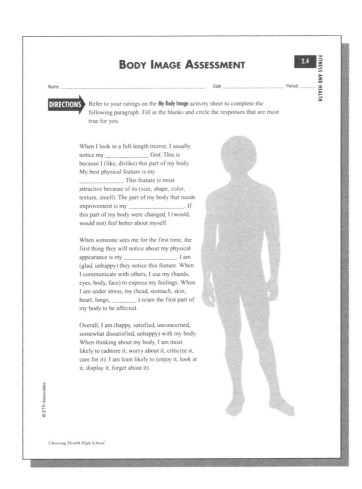

BODY IMAGE ASSESSMENT   2.4

Name _____ Date _____ Period _____

DIRECTIONS ▶ Refer to your ratings on the **My Body Image** activity sheet to complete the following paragraph. Fill in the blanks and circle the responses that are most true for you.

When I look in a full-length mirror, I usually notice my _____ first. This is because I (like, dislike) this part of my body. My best physical feature is my _____. This feature is most attractive because of its (size, shape, color, texture, smell). The part of my body that needs improvement is my _____. If this part of my body were changed, I (would, would not) feel better about myself.

When someone sees me for the first time, the first thing they will notice about my physical appearance is my _____. I am (glad, unhappy) they notice this feature. When I communicate with others, I use my (hands, eyes, body, face) to express my feelings. When I am under stress, my (head, stomach, skin, heart, lungs, _____) is/are the first part of my body to be affected.

Overall, I am (happy, satisfied, unconcerned, somewhat dissatisfied, unhappy) with my body. When thinking about my body, I am most likely to (admire it, worry about it, criticize it, care for it). I am least likely to (enjoy it, look at it, display it, forget about it).

© ETR Associates

Choosing Health High School

4. CHANGING YOUR BODY IMAGE

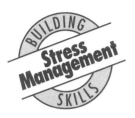

A BRAINSTORMING ACTIVITY

10 minutes

MATERIALS

◆ completed My Body Image (2.1) from Activity 1

Brainstorm reasons to change body image

Conduct a brainstorming session to identify reasons to change body image. Possible responses:

- Body image affects the way you feel about yourself.
- People with a positive body image are more confident.
- Improving body image will improve interactions with others.
- A positive body image will help you feel more comfortable living in your body.
- You are more likely to take care of your body if you feel good about it.
- Negative feelings about your body are stressful

Brainstorm ways to enhance body image

Conduct a brainstorming session to identify ways to enhance body image. Possible responses:

- Accept the features you cannot change.
- Work to alter the features you can change through personal behavior.
- Focus on the features you like.

(continued...)

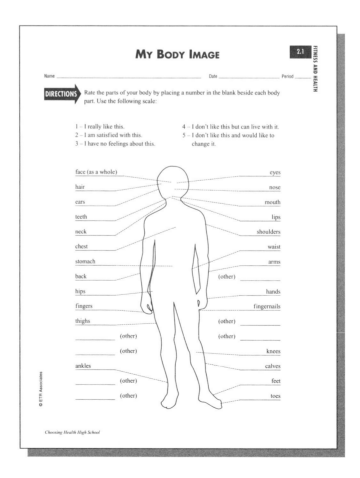

4. CHANGING YOUR BODY IMAGE

(CONTINUED)

Students identify physical features they like

Ask students to look again at the **My Body Image** activity sheet. Have them draw stars by the parts of their bodies they rated 1 and 2, the features they like. Why do they think these features are attractive? Ask students to answer the following questions either mentally or in writing. They should write down any conclusions.

- Have you always liked the features you starred?
- If so, why?
- If not, when did you change your mind? Why?
- Write a conclusion you have made based on this activity.

Ask volunteers to share general conclusions. Discourage specific examples or disclosures.

SHARPEN THE SKILL

STRESS MANAGEMENT—POSITIVE SELF-TALK

An important aspect of stress management is positive self-talk. Ask students to provide examples of positive self-talk statements they could say to themselves about body image.

---

5. ENHANCING OTHERS' BODY IMAGE

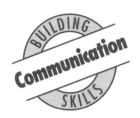

MATERIALS

♦ Partner Portrait (2.5)

A CLASS DISCUSSION ACTIVITY

Discuss compliments

Conduct a brief class discussion on giving and receiving compliments, using questions such as the following:

* How do you feel when someone compliments you on your appearance? (e.g., happy, proud, embarrassed)
* Is it easy or difficult for you to accept a compliment? Why or why not? (e.g., I'm not sure what to say. I feel that I don't deserve it. I don't want to seem conceited.)
* What is the best response to a compliment? (Express your thanks and allow yourself to accept the compliment.)

Students compliment partners

Have students choose partners with whom they feel comfortable and sit facing each other. Distribute the **Partner Portrait** activity sheet.

Ask students to read the example paragraph on the activity sheet, then portray one of their partner's most attractive features in writing or in a

(continued...)

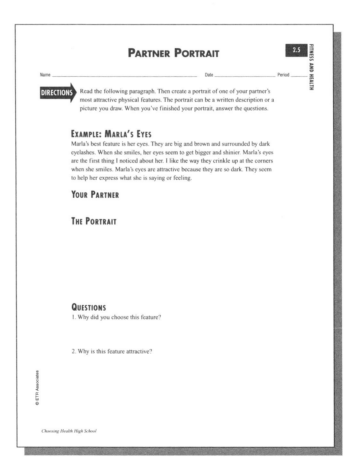

PARTNER PORTRAIT `2.5` FITNESS AND HEALTH

Name _____ Date _____ Period _____

DIRECTIONS Read the following paragraph. Then create a portrait of one of your partner's most attractive physical features. The portrait can be a written description or a picture you draw. When you've finished your portrait, answer the questions.

EXAMPLE: MARLA'S EYES
Marla's best feature is her eyes. They are big and brown and surrounded by dark eyelashes. When she smiles, her eyes seem to get bigger and shinier. Marla's eyes are the first thing I noticed about her. I like the way they crinkle up at the corners when she smiles. Marla's eyes are attractive because they are so dark. They seem to help her express what she is saying or feeling.

YOUR PARTNER

THE PORTRAIT

QUESTIONS
1. Why did you choose this feature?

2. Why is this feature attractive?

© ETR Associates

Choosing Health High School

5. ENHANCING OTHERS' BODY IMAGE

picture. When students have finished their portraits, they should answer the questions on the activity sheet. Emphasize that students should be sincere and sensitive in completing the portraits and answering the questions.

Students share responses

Ask students to take turns sharing their responses with each other. Remind students that the best way to receive a compliment is simply to say thank you. Suggest that students allow themselves to accept what was said.

SHARPEN THE SKILL
COMMUNICATION—GIVING COMPLIMENTS

Have students practice giving sincere compliments and notice the responses they get in return.

- Do most people "accept" the compliments?
- What kinds of responses do they get to the compliments?

EVALUATION

15 minutes

REVIEW

- Changing My Body Image *Example* (p. 27)

MATERIALS

- Changing My Body Image (2.6)

OBJECTIVE 1

Students will be able to:

Evaluate body image.

Distribute the **Changing My Body Image** evaluation sheet (Parts 1 and 2) and ask students to complete it. Remind students to describe *both* positive and negative aspects of their body image in Part 1. For Part 2, students may want to review their responses on the **My Body Image** activity sheet from Activity 1. In deciding how to answer the first question, they may choose a physical feature they disliked (rated 5) and want to change, or they may want to work to change the way they feel about the feature.

CRITERIA

Look for responses to be thoughtful and balanced. See the **Changing My Body Image** *Example* for evaluation criteria.

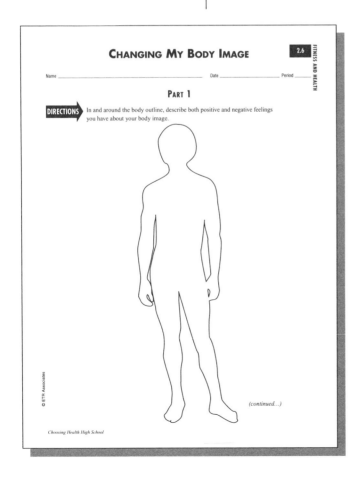

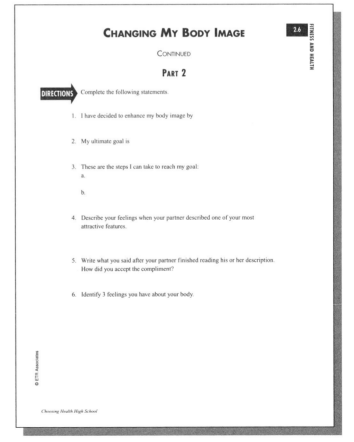

EVALUATION

OBJECTIVE 2

Students will be able to:

> **Demonstrate behaviors that enhance the body image of others.**

Ask 2 students to roleplay behaviors that enhance the body image of others. Give each volunteer a **Roleplay Card** and begin the roleplay. After the roleplay, ask the class to identify ways in which Tracy helped enhance Pat's body image.

CRITERIA

Look for student responses here and during Activity 5, the partner portrait activity, that demonstrate the ability to identify and deliver positive and sincere compliments.

10 minutes

MATERIALS

◆ prepared Roleplay Cards

MEETING STUDENT NEEDS

Take care in selecting roleplay participants. For example, select a "Pat" who feels good about his or her hair.

*

BODY IMAGE

The mental picture people have of their bodies is called "body image." Body image is part of self-esteem, or feelings about self.

Levels of self-esteem change based on daily experiences, as well as interpersonal experiences. How a person perceives his or her physical appearance and how a person's appearance is viewed by others influences self-esteem.

Our culture tends to rely heavily on appearance in making judgments and assumptions about an individual. Certain features (for example, a thin body) are glamorized at the expense of other body types. Sometimes our culture makes it difficult to feel good about our "less than perfect" bodies.

Each person is unique, with physical features that are a part of who she or he is as an individual. All people have features they dislike. Some of these features can be changed through personal behavior. Others cannot be changed.

During adolescence, physical characteristics change. Teens grow taller and heavier, skin and hair changes, voices become more mature and secondary sexual characteristics appear. It is not surprising that it may take time for adolescents to grow comfortable with all these changes.

Other people can affect a person's body image by what they say and how they react. Adolescents may be particularly sensitive to how their peers perceive them. Sincere compliments may help a person feel good about his or her physical self. Recognition and acceptance of each individual's physical appearance creates an atmosphere that fosters the development of a positive body image.

CHANGING MY BODY IMAGE

EXAMPLE

PART 1

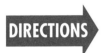 In and around the body outline, describe both positive and negative feelings you have about your body image.

Descriptions should include both features that are viewed positively and features viewed negatively. Examples:

- *My nose is great because it's just like my grandmother's.*

- *My hair is a big problem because it is so oily.*

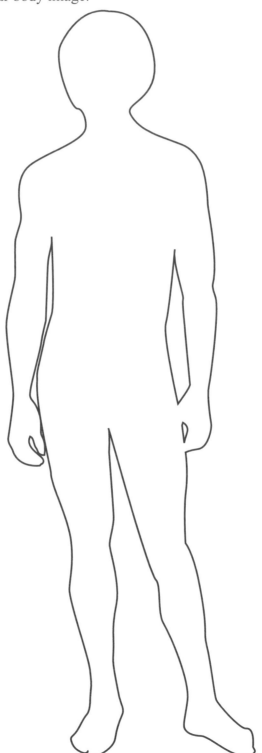

(continued...)

EXAMPLE, CONTINUED

PART 2

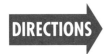 Complete the following statements.

1. I have decided to enhance my body image by
   changing the way I feel about my hair.

2. My ultimate goal is
   to feel proud of the way I look.

3. These are the steps I can take to reach my goal:
   a. **Go to a stylist and get a new haircut.**

   b. **Think about what I like about my hair (the color) instead of what I don't like.**

4. Describe your feelings when your partner described one of your most attractive features.
   A little embarrassed, but mostly pleased that someone noticed my dimples.

5. Write what you said after your partner finished reading his or her description. How did you accept the compliment?
   "Thanks, I appreciate what you said."

6. Identify 3 feelings you have about your body.
   happy
   curious
   concerned

ON YOUR MARK, GET SET, GO!

TIME

2 periods

ACTIVITIES

1. Assessing Aerobic Capacity

2. Assessing Body Composition

3. Assessing Flexibility

4. Assessing Muscular Strength and Endurance

5. Assessing Fitness

ON YOUR MARK, GET SET, GO!

OBJECTIVE

Students will be able to:

> **Analyze their individual levels of fitness.**

GETTING STARTED

Copy for each student:

- Assess Your Fitness (3.1)

Make transparency of:

- How Fit Are You? (3.2)

SPECIAL STEPS

Remind students to wear appropriate clothing and shoes for each activity:

- Activity 1—running shoes
- Activity 2—shorts and T-shirts
- Activities 3 and 4—comfortable, loose clothing

Build Sit and Reach Apparatus. See Activity 3 (p. 34).
Gather materials and prepare for fitness assessments. See
Activity 1 (p. 32), Activity 2 (p. 33) and Activity 4 (p. 35).

UNIT OVERVIEW

PURPOSE

If they are to make choices that enhance their physical health, students must be aware of their personal level of fitness. Assessment of students' aerobic capacity, body composition, flexibility, muscular strength and endurance provides the foundation for realistic and regular exercise patterns.

MAIN POINTS

* An individual's level of fitness can be determined by assessing the elements of fitness.
* Specific activities provide measurements of the elements of fitness.

REVIEW

To increase your understanding of fitness assessments, review **Conducting the Personal Fitness Assessments** *Instant Expert* (p. 38).

VOCABULARY

cool-down—A gradual decrease from vigorous exercise.

skin-fold measurements—A method for measuring body composition that uses calipers to measure the thickness of folds of skin.

warm-up—The first portion of a workout, designed to prepare the body for vigorous exercise.

1. ASSESSING AEROBIC CAPACITY

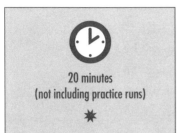

20 minutes
(not including practice runs)

MATERIALS

♦ A stopwatch or watch with a second hand

♦ A 440-yard or 400-meter track, or any other flat, measured area that will provide a distance of 1 mile

♦ Assess Your Fitness (3.1)

MEETING STUDENT NEEDS

If given a choice, some students may choose not to participate in all or some of the assessments. You may make this lesson elective or set up alternative times in order to assess students with complete privacy. However, all students should be encouraged to participate as fully as possible. Be sure that students with known medical conditions that would contraindicate vigorous exercise do not take the tests. Modification of some assessment activities may be indicated for some students who are physically challenged.

Students prepare for 1-mile walk/run

Allow students to participate in 2 or 3 practice runs. Emphasize the concept of pace. Results are better if students maintain a constant pace during most of the test, walking only if necessary. Have students engage in warm-up activities such as stretching, walking and jogging before the test.

Students walk/run

Have students run 1 mile in their fastest possible time, beginning on the signal, "Ready, start." As students cross the finish line, call the elapsed time.

Students cool down

Have students engage in cool-down activities such as walking and stretching after the run.

Students record scores

Distribute the Assess Your Fitness activity sheet and have students write down their time for the run.

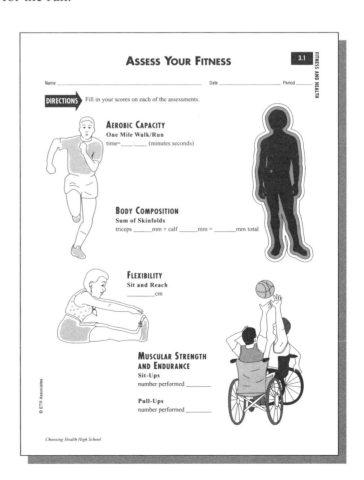

2. ASSESSING BODY COMPOSITION

Assess students' body composition

For the measurement, have each student stand erect with the right arm relaxed and the palm facing the leg. Measure the triceps skinfold midway between the elbow and the shoulder.

Have the student place the right foot on a bench with the knee flexed. Measure the calf skinfold on the inside of the lower right leg. Measure each skinfold site 3 consecutive times and record the middle (median) score. Add the calf and triceps skinfolds to determine the final score. (Example: reading 1 = 10cm, reading 2 = 12cm, reading 3 = 10cm. Record 10cm.)

Students record scores

Have students write their final scores on the **Assess Your Fitness** activity sheet.

2–3 minutes per student

✸

MATERIALS
- Skinfold calipers
- Assess Your Fitness (3.1)

✸

MEASURING SKINFOLDS

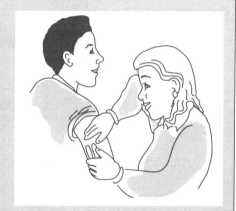

Triceps

❶ Skinfold should be measured halfway between the elbow and shoulder.

❷ Grasp and lift the skinfold with your thumb and index finger, 1/2 inch above the midpoint of the arm.

❸ Place the calipers below your finger, at the midpoint of the arm.

Calf

❶ Skinfold should be measured at the largest part of the calf.

❷ Grasp and lift the skinfold with your thumb and index finger, slightly above the widest part of the calf.

❸ Place the calipers below your finger at the level of the widest part of the calf.

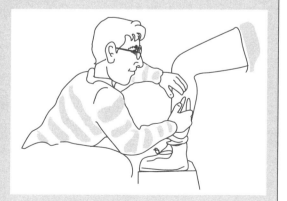

3. Assessing Flexibility

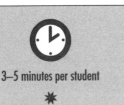

3–5 minutes per student

MATERIALS

- Assess Your Fitness (3.1)

SIT AND REACH APPARATUS

- wooden box or bench
- meter stick
- small nails or strong tape

MEETING STUDENT NEEDS

Coordinate assessments with persons who are qualified to conduct assessments for students who are physically challenged.

Students warm up

Have students warm up by performing 2–3 slow, sustained stretches of the low back and posterior thighs.

Measure students' flexibility

As students are tested, have them remove their shoes and sit in front of the apparatus with legs fully extended and feet shoulder-width apart. Have a monitor place his or her hands lightly across the knees to prevent flexing during the test. The feet should be flat against the end of the box or bench and the arms extended forward with the hands on top of each other.

Have the student reach forward, with the palms down, along the measuring scale 4 times, holding the position of maximum reach on the fourth time. The position must be held for 1 second. Repeat the test if the hands reach out unevenly or the knees flex during the trial.

Students record scores

Have students write their distance of maximum reach on the **Assess Your Fitness** activity sheet.

SIT AND REACH APPARATUS

1 Gather materials.

2 Position the box or bench with a flat surface perpendicular to the floor, for students' feet to rest against.

3 Place the meter stick along top surface of the box or bench, with the 23cm mark even with the edge where the students' feet will be placed. The 0cm mark should be closest to the student.

4 Nail or securely tape the meter stick in place.

5 Place the apparatus against a wall or other immovable object to keep it from moving away from students during the test.

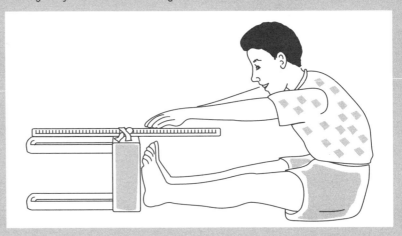

4. ASSESSING MUSCULAR STRENGTH AND ENDURANCE

Explain how to perform sit-ups

Assign each student a partner. Have one student from each pair lie on his or her back with knees flexed and feet on the floor. The heels should be between 12 and 18 inches from the buttocks, the arms crossed on the chest, with the hands on the opposite shoulders. Remind students to keep the chin tucked toward the chest. Partners hold the feet to keep them on the floor.

Explain that to perform a sit-up, the student should tighten the abdominal muscles to curl into the sitting position. The sit-up is completed when the student returns to the down position (the midback makes contact with the floor or mat) after touching the thighs with the elbows. Tell students they may rest between sit-ups; but the objective is to perform as many sit-ups as possible in 60 seconds.

Students perform sit-ups

Have students begin the sit-ups on the signal "Ready, go" and perform as many sit-ups as possible in 60 seconds. Ask the partners to count the sit-ups. After 60 seconds, signal students to "stop." The number of sit-ups performed correctly in 60 seconds is the score. Have students switch partners, and repeat the test.

Note: Sit-ups can be performed as a group as described, or you can assess students individually.

Students perform pull-ups

To begin the test, have the student hang from the bar with his or her arms fully extended. The feet should not touch the floor, and an overhand grip should be used. From the hanging position, have the student raise his or her body until the chin is over the bar. The student should perform as many correctly executed pull-ups as possible. There is no time limit.

To ensure students' safety, be sure the bar is securely attached. Have someone "spot" students as they perform the pull-ups.

Students record scores

Have students write their scores on the **Assess Your Fitness** activity sheet.

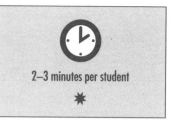

2–3 minutes per student

✳

MATERIALS

♦ mats or other comfortable surfaces

♦ stopwatch or watch with a second hand

♦ metal or wooden bar approximately 1-1/2 inch in diameter, hung high enough off the floor so that students' feet will not touch.

♦ Assess Your Fitness (3.1)

MEETING STUDENT NEEDS

The physical abilities and fitness levels of students vary. Students who cannot perform a pull-up often find their fitness levels improve with exercise.

5. ASSESSING FITNESS

15 minutes

MATERIALS

◆ completed Assess Your Fitness (3.1)

◆ transparency of How Fit Are You? (3.2)

MEETING STUDENT NEEDS

Emphasize that the purpose of these activities was for students to discover their own level of fitness, not to compete with others. Discourage any disclosure of specific scores.

Students review scores

Ask students to take out the Assess Your Fitness activity sheet and look over their scores for the fitness assessments.

Students assess fitness

Display the How Fit Are You? transparency and ask students to compare their scores on each of the fitness assessments with the fitness measurements listed on the transparency. Ask students to put a star by the element of fitness that was best for them. Ask them to circle the element they most need to improve. On the back of the activity sheet, have students describe strategies they can use to improve their level of fitness.

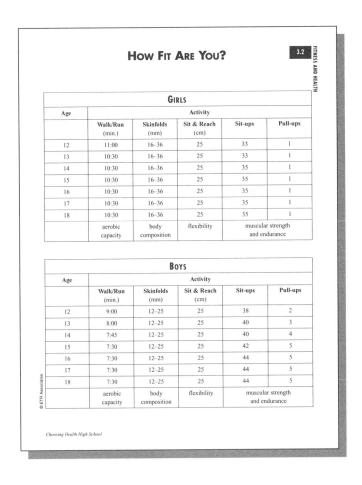

HOW FIT ARE YOU? | 3.2 | FITNESS AND HEALTH

GIRLS					
Age	Activity				
	Walk/Run (min.)	Skinfolds (mm)	Sit & Reach (cm)	Sit-ups	Pull-ups
12	11:00	16–36	25	33	1
13	10:30	16–36	25	33	1
14	10:30	16–36	25	35	1
15	10:30	16–36	25	35	1
16	10:30	16–36	25	35	1
17	10:30	16–36	25	35	1
18	10:30	16–36	25	35	1
	aerobic capacity	body composition	flexibility	muscular strength and endurance	

BOYS					
Age	Activity				
	Walk/Run (min.)	Skinfolds (mm)	Sit & Reach (cm)	Sit-ups	Pull-ups
12	9:00	12–25	25	38	2
13	8:00	12–25	25	40	3
14	7:45	12–25	25	40	4
15	7:30	12–25	25	42	5
16	7:30	12–25	25	44	5
17	7:30	12–25	25	44	5
18	7:30	12–25	25	44	5
	aerobic capacity	body composition	flexibility	muscular strength and endurance	

© ETR Associates

Choosing Health High School

EVALUATION

OBJECTIVE

Students will be able to:

> **Analyze their individual levels of fitness.**

Observe students throughout the assessments to assess their level of participation and their ability to demonstrate each activity. Review the **Assess Your Fitness** activity sheet for student scores for each of the fitness activities. Look to see which areas of fitness students analyzed as high and as low and review the strategies they listed to improve their fitness.

CRITERIA

Walking/running the mile in less time, reaching farther on the sit and reach and performing more sit-ups or pull-ups indicates a higher level of fitness for each element. Students' descriptions of how to improve their level of fitness should correlate to the lower score areas. Students who exceed the range on skinfold measurements can reduce their risk of health problems by decreasing the amount of fatty foods they eat and exercising more.

MATERIALS

♦ completed Assess Your Fitness (3.1)

CONDUCTING THE PERSONAL FITNESS ASSESSMENTS

It is easier to move students through all activities in 1 or 2 class periods if you divide the class into groups and move students through the assessments in a round-robin fashion.

Set up a station for each of the 5 assessments. Enlist the help of students or other teachers to serve as supervisors for each of the stations. Some students may be sensitive about their performance on the assessments. Ask supervisors to encourage participation, but emphasize the importance of being sensitive to students' feelings. Students with known medical problems that would contraindicate vigorous exercise should *not* take the tests.

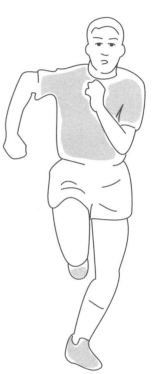

AEROBIC CAPACITY

A 1-mile walk/run can be used to check aerobic capacity. For this assessment you will need to have access to a 440-yard or 400-meter track, or any other flat, measured area that will provide a distance of 1 mile.

Students should be encouraged to run as far as possible, but allowed to walk if necessary. Be sure students warm up before the activity and cool down after it. For example, students could walk 1 lap before and after the activity.

BODY COMPOSITION

A sum of skinfold measurements can be used to assess body composition. Skinfold calipers are used to take these measurements. A variety of calipers are available. Good results are possible with inexpensive plastic calipers if they are used correctly. Calipers should produce a constant pressure of 10 grams per square millimeter.

(continued...)

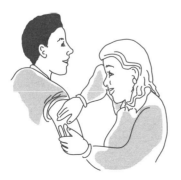

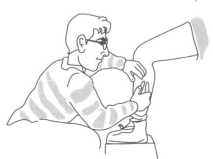

CONDUCTING THE PERSONAL FITNESS ASSESSMENTS

INSTANT EXPERT

FLEXIBILITY

A sit and reach apparatus with a centimeter measuring scale can be used to assess flexibility. The apparatus must be placed against an immovable object, such as a wall, to prevent it from moving away from the student during the test.

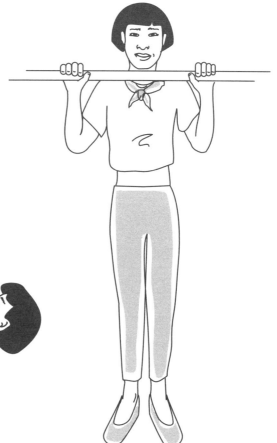

MUSCULAR STRENGTH AND ENDURANCE

Sit-ups and pull-ups are used to measure muscular strength and endurance. During sit-ups, the heels should be placed 12–18 inches from the buttocks. Sit-ups should always be performed with bent legs. Be sure students are doing sit-ups correctly.

For pull-ups, check to make sure students use an overhand grip and begin the pull-up with extended arms. One pull-up has been executed when the chin is over the bar.

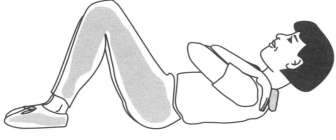

In a Heartbeat

TIME

2 periods

ACTIVITIES

1. Improving Aerobic Capacity

2. An Aerobic Workout

3. Personal Plan

IN A HEARTBEAT

OBJECTIVE

Students will be able to:

> Synthesize a plan to improve aerobic capacity.

GETTING STARTED

Have:

- stopwatch or watch with a second hand

Make transparency of:

- Aerobic Prescription (4.1)
- Your Target Heart Rate (4.2)
- Personal Plan Example (4.3)

Copy for each student:

- Your Target Heart Rate (4.2)
- Personal Plan (4.4)

SPECIAL STEPS

Ask students to wear clothing and shoes for exercising.
Optional: Have cassettes of popular music and cassette player
   or an aerobic dance video and video cassette player. See
   Activity 2.

UNIT OVERVIEW

PURPOSE

When students understand ways to improve their aerobic capacity, they are more motivated to engage in regular aerobic activities. By participating in an aerobic workout, students may be encouraged to engage in exercise programs geared to their own interests and abilities.

MAIN POINTS

✳ Aerobic capacity can be increased through regular participation in activities that place demands on the heart and lungs.

✳ Activities that increase aerobic capacity involve continuous and repetitive movements of large muscle groups.

✳ Aerobic activities should be performed for at least 20 minutes at the target heart rate, 3–6 times per week.

REVIEW

To increase your understanding of aerobic capacity, review **Improving Aerobic Capacity Instant Expert** (p. 49).

VOCABULARY

aerobic activity—Exercise that involves continuous and repetitive movements of the large muscle groups; e.g., jogging, bicycling, skating, cross country skiing, walking and jumping rope.

frequency—The number of times an action is repeated in a given period.

intensity—A higher-than-normal level of stress that is self-imposed during exercising.

stretching—Activities designed to loosen connective tissue (tendons and ligaments) and muscles.

target heart rate—Figure used to determine the number of heartbeats per minute required to improve aerobic capacity.

time—A period during which an action takes place.

1. IMPROVING AEROBIC CAPACITY

25 minutes

MATERIALS

- transparency of Aerobic Prescription (4.1)
- transparency of Your Target Heart Rate (4.2)
- Your Target Heart Rate (4.2)
- stopwatch or watch with a second hand

MEETING STUDENT NEEDS

The THR calculation may not apply to students who are taking certain medications or are obese. As a general rule, students should exercise at an intensity level that causes them to breathe harder but still be able to carry on a conversation during exercise. While it is important to assist students with special needs separately, it is also important to do it in a way that does not call attention to differences. Sensitivity and discretion are key.

Discuss aerobic capacity

Display the **Aerobic Prescription** transparency. Discuss aerobic capacity, using the **Improving Aerobic Capacity** *Instant Expert* as a guide.

(continued...)

AEROBIC PRESCRIPTION `4.1` FITNESS AND HEALTH

Frequency—3 to 6 Times Each Week
Intensity—At Your Target Heart Rate
Time—At Least 20 Minutes
Type of Activity—Continuous and Repetitive

Some Popular Aerobic Activities

aerobic dance	skateboarding	swimming
ballet	skating	tennis
basketball	skiing	volleyball
bicycling	soccer	walking
gymnastics		
jogging		
jumping rope		
karate		
racquetball		
rowing		

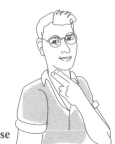

Checking Your Pulse

© ETR Associates

Choosing Health High School

---

1. IMPROVING AEROBIC CAPACITY

CONTINUED

Calculate target heart rates

Show students the transparency of **Your Target Heart Rate**. Explain how to calculate target heart rate, using the **Improving Aerobic Capacity** *Instant Expert* as a guide. Fill in the transparency for yourself or a hypothetical student to demonstrate.

Distribute the **Your Target Heart Rate** activity sheet. Have students sit quietly and find their pulse. Time students for 15 seconds as they count the beats. Have them multiply by 4 to find their resting heart rates. Then have students calculate their target heart rates using the formula on the activity sheet.

> ### EXTEND THE LEARNING
> Have students calculate the number of heart beats increased aerobic capacity can save. A highly trained athlete's heart may beat only 40 times per minute, while the average heart rate is 75 beats per minute. In 1 year, how many more times than the athlete's will the average person's heart beat?
> Answer: 18,396,000 times
> (The average person's heart will beat 39,420,000 times. The athlete's will beat 21,024,000 times.)
>

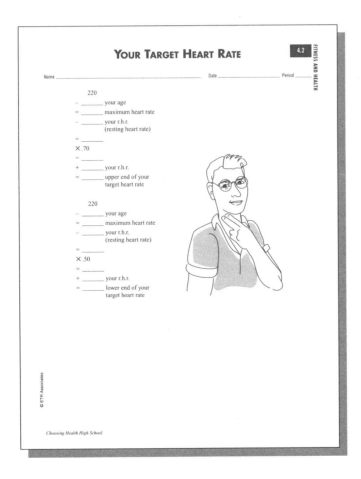

2. AN AEROBIC WORKOUT

40 minutes

✳

MATERIALS

♦ *Optional:* cassettes of popular music and cassette player or an aerobic dance video and VCR

✳

MEETING STUDENT NEEDS

Some students may be unable to perform all the steps or continue activity for 20 minutes. It is more important to continue moving than to perform the steps correctly. Emphasize the importance of exercising at a comfortable pace.

✳

Students warm up

Begin the workout by having students jog slowly for about 5 minutes to warm up. Then have students perform stretching exercises for about 5 minutes. (See the Exercises for Flexibility section of the Improving Body Composition and Flexibility *Instant Expert* in Unit 5, p. 60.)

Students practice aerobic workout

Have students jog or dance to reach their target heart rates (THR). Students should continue the activity for at least 20 minutes. At 5 minute intervals have students check their pulse while you time them for 6 seconds. Students can add a zero to the 6-second count to get their current heart rate and determine whether they have reached or are maintaining their THR.

Students cool down

Guide students to reduce their activity over a 5-minute period to cool down. Conclude the workout by having students perform the stretching exercises again.

Ongoing Assessment Look for student progress in aerobic capacity. This will be generally demonstrated by lower heart rates and the ability to sustain activity.

3. PERSONAL PLAN

A PERSONAL CONTRACT ACTIVITY

Discuss planning

Display the **Personal Plan Example** transparency. Explain the importance of setting realistic and measurable goals for improving or maintaining aerobic capacity. Planning is an important step in any exercise program. For each step in the plan, students need to consider what type of activity best suits them.

Develop plans

Distribute the **Personal Plan** activity sheet and have students write a personal plan for improving or maintaining aerobic capacity. The plan should include a choice(s) of aerobic activities and an aerobic exercise plan (including warm-up, stretching, exercise at the THR, cool-down and stretching).

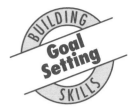

15 minutes

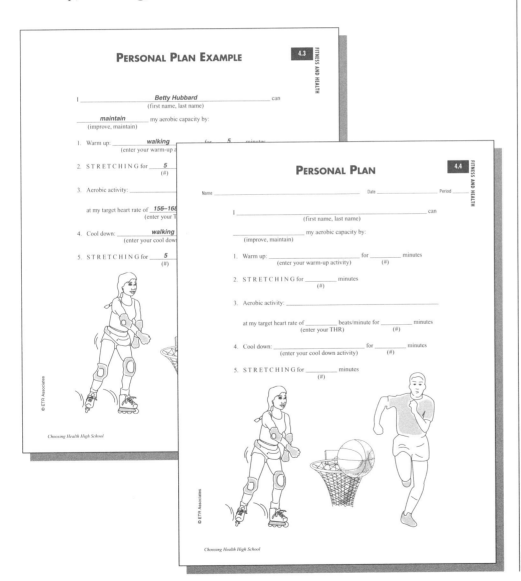

MATERIALS

♦ transparency of Personal Plan Example (4.3)
♦ Personal Plan (4.4)

SHARPEN THE SKILL
GOAL SETTING—PAMPHLETS AND POSTERS

Have students work in pairs or triads to develop pamphlets or posters that identify a goal and describe activities that can improve aerobic capacity. Students can outline the components and steps of an aerobic workout. They can use pictures from magazines or their own drawings to illustrate the pamphlets or posters.

EVALUATION

OBJECTIVE

Students will be able to:

> **Synthesize a plan to improve aerobic capacity.**

CRITERIA

Review students' **Personal Plan** activity sheets. Look for completeness and appropriateness of student plans, based on their personal levels of aerobic fitness. Plans should include:

- a warm-up, stretching, aerobic, cool-down and stretching component
- exercise at target heart rate

See the **Improving Aerobic Capacity** *Instant Expert* for evaluation criteria.

IMPROVING AEROBIC CAPACITY

Activities that improve aerobic capacity must be of a certain type, and fulfill the requirements for frequency, intensity and time (FIT).

TYPE OF ACTIVITY

The exercise should be continuous and involve repetitive movements of the large muscle groups. Swimming, cycling, basketball, cross-country skiing, aerobic dancing, walking and jogging meet this requirement. Other activities such as tennis and racquetball can qualify if the action is continuous. Whichever exercise is used, an aerobic workout should follow the same pattern:

1. Warm up to elevate body temperature (5 minutes).
2. Stretch to loosen connective tissues and muscles to prevent injury (5–10 minutes).
3. Exercise at target heart rate (at least 20 minutes).
4. Cool down by moving more slowly (5 minutes).
5. Stretch to prevent muscle soreness (5–10 minutes).

IMPROVING AEROBIC CAPACITY

Improvement in aerobic capacity can be achieved through many activities, as long as the activity places sufficient demand on the heart and lungs. The acronym FIT—frequency, intensity, time—provides a basis for evaluating activities.

Frequency—To improve aerobic capacity, you must exercise 3–4 times per week.

Intensity—Activities should be performed with enough intensity to reach and maintain target heart rate (THR).

Time—Exercise at the THR should be maintained for 20–30 minutes.

TARGET HEART RATE

Target heart rate (THR) is used to monitor aerobic capacity. The THR is the number of times the heart needs to beat each minute to have a positive effect on the cardiorespiratory system. To determine THR, use the following formula:

- Subtract your age from 220 to find your maximum heart rate.
- Subtract your resting heart rate—the number of times your heart beats when you are at rest—from your maximum heart rate and multiply by 70%.
- Add this figure to your resting heart rate to find the upper end of your target heart rate.
- To find the lower end of your target heart rate, repeat the process, but multiply by 50%.

(continued...)

IMPROVING AEROBIC CAPACITY

For example, the THR for a person who is 16 years old and has a resting heart rate of 73 beats per minute would be calculated as follows: $220 - 16 = 204 - 73 = 131 \times .50 = 65.5 + 73 = 138.5$ (lower end of the range) $220 - 16 = 204 - 73 = 131 \times .70 = 91.7 + 73 = 164.7$ (upper end of the range). While exercising, this 16 year old's heart should beat between 139 and 154 beats per minute. (Students between the ages of 13 and 20 have a THR of between 135 and 168 beats per minute.)

To find your target heart rate while exercising, stop your activity and find your pulse at the carotid artery. Once you have found your pulse, count the number of beats you feel in a 6-second period and add a zero. This number will be your heart rate. If this heart rate is below your THR, you need to exercise harder. If this heart rate is above your THR, you need to exercise with less intensity.

LOOKING GOOD— FEELING GOOD

TIME

1–2 periods

ACTIVITIES

1. Improving Flexibility

2. Improving Strength and Endurance

3. How to Get Fit

4. Fitness Facilities

LOOKING GOOD—
FEELING GOOD

OBJECTIVES

Students will be able to:

> 1. Analyze ways to improve body composition, flexibility, muscular strength and endurance.

> 2. Analyze fitness facilities or programs in the community.

GETTING STARTED

Make transparency of:

- Exercises for Flexibility (5.1)
- Exercises for Muscular Strength and Endurance (5.3)

Copy for each student:

- Improving Flexibility (5.2)
- Improving Strength and Endurance (5.4)
- Fitness Focus (5.5)
- Facility or Program Survey (5.6)

SPECIAL STEPS

Ask students to wear clothing and shoes for exercising. Have exercise mats or other comfortable surfaces available.

UNIT OVERVIEW

PURPOSE

Maintaining a healthful body composition, an appropriate degree of flexibility, and an adequate level of muscular strength and endurance enables people to meet the demands of daily living and reduces the risk of injury. This lesson encourages students to explore ways in which these elements of fitness can be enhanced.

MAIN POINTS

* Body composition is influenced by activity level and eating habits.
* Flexibility can be improved through stretching exercises.
* Free weights, weight machines and calisthenics can improve muscular strength and endurance.
* The community has resources that promote fitness.

REVIEW

To increase your understanding of exercises to increase flexibility and muscle strength and endurance, review Improving Body Composition and Flexibility *Instant Expert* (p. 60) and Improving Muscular Strength and Endurance *Instant Expert* (p. 64).

VOCABULARY

calisthenics—Exercises done without equipment; e.g., pushups, sit-ups.

complex carbohydrates—A source of vitamins, minerals and energy; found in whole grains, fruits and vegetables.

fat—A nutrient that is a source of energy and that can be stored.

free weights—Hand-held weights, barbells and dumbbells.

overloading—To demand more work from muscles than is normally required.

rep (repetition)—Each time an exercise movement is completed.

set—Group(s) of repetitions.

weight machines—Equipment designed to increase muscular strength and endurance.

1. Improving Flexibility

25 minutes

MATERIALS

- transparency of Exercises for Flexibility (5.1)
- Improving Flexibility (5.2)

Discuss how to improve body composition

Present guidelines for improving body composition through good nutrition and exercise, using the **Improving Body Composition and Flexibility** *Instant Expert* as a guide.

Discuss flexibility

Present the benefits of stretching and explain the guidelines for safe stretching, using the **Improving Body Composition and Flexibility** *Instant Expert* as a guide.

Students perform exercises

Display the **Exercises for Flexibility** transparency. Explain and demonstrate each exercise, using the **Improving Body Composition and Flexibility** *Instant Expert* as a guide. Have students perform each exercise after you explain it. Distribute the **Improving Flexibility** activity sheet. Tell students to keep this sheet as a guide.

Ongoing Assessment Assess students' ability to perform the exercises correctly. See the Exercises for Flexibility section of the **Improving Body Composition and Flexibility** *Instant Expert* for criteria.

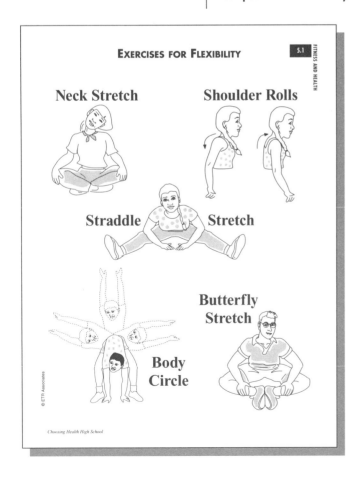

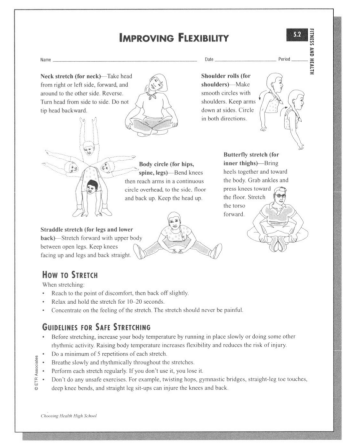

2. IMPROVING STRENGTH AND ENDURANCE

(A DEMONSTRATION ACTIVITY)

Discuss muscular strength and endurance

Present the basic concepts of weight training and calisthenics, using the Improving Muscular Strength and Endurance *Instant Expert* as a guide.

Students perform exercises

Display the Exercises for Muscular Strength and Endurance transparency. Explain and demonstrate each exercise, using the Improving Muscular Strength and Endurance *Instant Expert* as a guide. Have students perform each exercise after you explain it. Distribute the Improving Strength and Endurance activity sheet. Tell students to keep this sheet as a guide to working out at home.

Ongoing Assessment) Assess students' ability to perform the exercises correctly. See the Exercises for Muscular Strength and Endurance section of the Improving Muscular Strength and Endurance *Instant Expert* for criteria.

25 minutes

MATERIALS

♦ transparency of Exercises for Muscular Strength and Endurance (5.3)

♦ Improving Strength and Endurance (5.4)

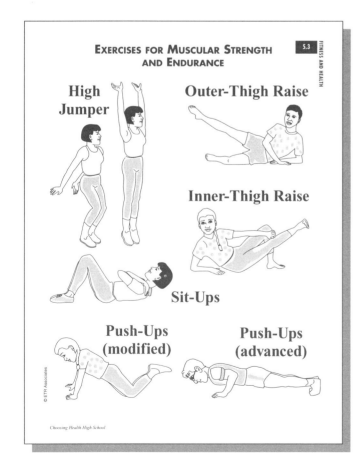

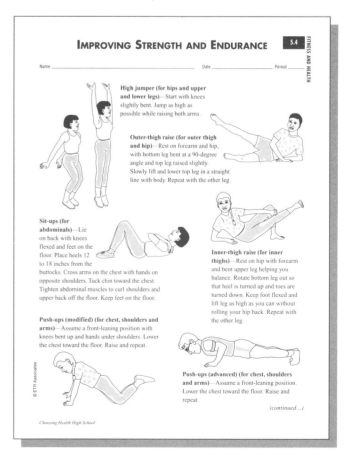

3. How to Get Fit

25 minutes

MATERIALS

◆ Fitness Focus (5.5)

Groups discuss exercise

Divide the class into groups of 3–4. Distribute the **Fitness Focus** activity sheet. Explain the group assignment:

- Read and discuss the case studies.
- Write an exercise prescription that would enable each person to improve his or her element of fitness. List specific ways in which the element of fitness can be improved.
- Prepare to explain or demonstrate your prescription for 1 of the case studies.

Groups report

Have each group explain or demonstrate its recommendations for at least 1 of the people in the case studies. This may include demonstrations of activities or exercises.

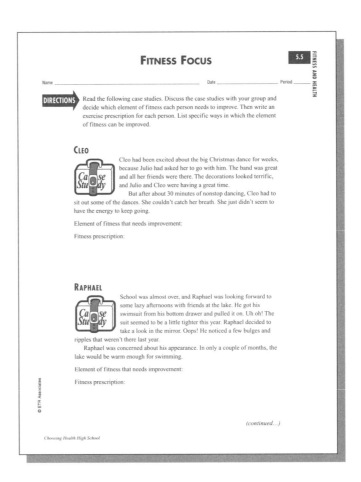

4. FITNESS FACILITIES

Groups research fitness facilities or programs

Divide the class into small groups and distribute the **Facility or Program Survey** activity sheet. Explain the group assignment:

- Choose a local public or private fitness facility or program to research. Look in the phone book under Health Clubs or contact local schools or colleges, community centers, parks and fitness organizations. Many communities send out catalogs of recreational programs. Check to see if your community has a recreation program.
- Make arrangements to visit or call the facility or program and research the activities it offers. Answer all the questions on the activity sheet.
- Prepare a report on the facility or program to present to the class.

(continued...)

10 minutes, plus 55 minutes
for reports and discussion

❈

MATERIALS

♦ Facility or Program Survey (5.6)

❈

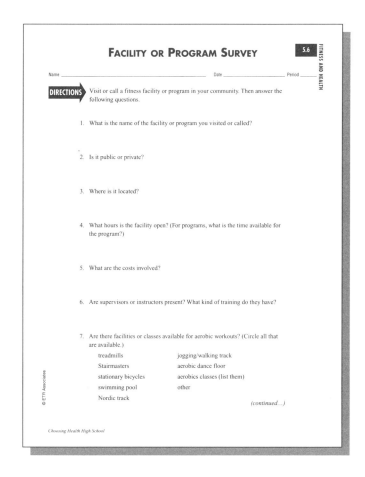

FACILITY OR PROGRAM SURVEY | 5.6 | FITNESS AND HEALTH

Name _____ Date _____ Period _____

DIRECTIONS Visit or call a fitness facility or program in your community. Then answer the following questions.

1. What is the name of the facility or program you visited or called?

2. Is it public or private?

3. Where is it located?

4. What hours is the facility open? (For programs, what is the time available for the program?)

5. What are the costs involved?

6. Are supervisors or instructors present? What kind of training do they have?

7. Are there facilities or classes available for aerobic workouts? (Circle all that are available.)

treadmills	jogging/walking track
Stairmasters	aerobic dance floor
stationary bicycles	aerobics classes (list them)
swimming pool	other
Nordic track	

(continued...)

© ETR Associates

Choosing Health High School

4. FITNESS FACILITIES

$$\text{CONTINUED}$$

COMMUNITY LINK

Be sure to coordinate student efforts, so a variety of facilities are covered and no single facility or program is deluged with student calls or visits. Encourage students to investigate both public and private facilities and programs.

Groups report

Have groups report their findings. As a class, evaluate the quality of facilities and programs available in your community. Analyze reasons why people choose one facility or program over another. These may include:

- availability
- cost
- social aspects
- fun/enjoyment
- fitness benefits—aerobic capacity, body composition, flexibility, muscular strength and endurance

- variety of activities
- variety of equipment
- location

EVALUATION

OBJECTIVE 1

Students will be able to:

> **Analyze ways to improve body composition, flexibility, muscular strength and endurance.**

Review the **Fitness Focus** activity sheets and observe students' work in small groups and group presentations to assess their ability to analyze ways to improve fitness.

CRITERIA

See the **Fitness Focus** *Key* for evaluation criteria.

REVIEW

◆ Fitness Focus *Key* (p. 66)

MATERIALS

◆ completed Fitness Focus (5.5), from Activity 3

OBJECTIVE 2

Students will be able to:

> **Analyze fitness facilities or programs in the community.**

Review students' **Facility or Program Survey** activity sheets and assess group reports for students' ability to analyze fitness facilities and programs.

CRITERIA

Look for groups to note desirability of facilities or programs that:

- provide an aerobic component
- are accessible (location, hours, cost)
- monitor participants' fitness level
- are staffed by qualified personnel
- encourage regular participation
- provide classes/equipment that are enjoyable to students

MATERIALS

◆ completed Facility or Program Survey (5.6), from Activity 4

IMPROVING BODY COMPOSITION AND FLEXIBILITY

BODY COMPOSITION

Body composition can be improved by making regular exercise and good nutrition a part of one's normal routine. The following are guidelines for good nutrition:

- Eat a variety of foods from the 5 basic food groups—meat/protein, fruits, vegetables, grains and dairy.
- Limit the amount of salt and refined sugar in the diet.
- Eat complex carbohydrates (fruits, vegetables and whole grain products).
- Avoid fad diets.
- Limit fatty foods (french fries, desserts and chips).

When muscles are used in regular exercise, they become stronger and firmer. Physical activity not only builds muscles—it also burns calories. Because exercise helps burn excess fat and build muscle, the person looks and feels better.

FLEXIBILITY

The body becomes more flexible if stretching is a part of one's daily activity. Stretching can:

- Help prevent injuries such as muscle strains and shin splints.
- Reduce muscle tension and promote relaxation.
- Serve as a warm-up for vigorous physical activities.

Static or sustained stretching is the safest way to stretch. When stretching:

- Reach to the point of discomfort, then back off slightly.
- Relax and hold the stretch for 10–20 seconds.
- Concentrate on the feeling. The stretch should never be painful.

GUIDELINES FOR SAFE STRETCHING

- Before stretching, increase body temperature by running in place slowly or doing some other rhythmic activity. This reduces the risk of injury.
- Do a minimum of 5 repetitions of each stretch.
- Breathe slowly and rhythmically throughout the stretches.
- Perform each stretch regularly. If you don't use it, you lose it.
- Don't do any unsafe exercises. For example, twisting hops, gymnastic bridges, straight-leg toe touches, deep knee bends, and straight leg sit-ups can injure the knees and back.

(continued...)

IMPROVING BODY COMPOSITION AND FLEXIBILITY

EXERCISES FOR FLEXIBILITY

The following stretches will increase flexibility.

Neck stretch (for neck)—Take head from right or left side, forward, and around to the other side. Reverse. Turn head from side to side. Do not tip head backward.

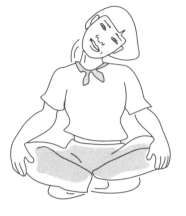

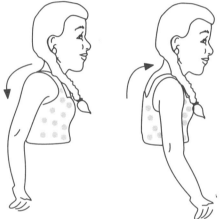

Shoulder rolls (for shoulders)—Make smooth circles with shoulders. Keep arms down at sides. Circle in both directions.

Body circle (for hips, spine, legs)—Bend knees then reach arms in a continuous circle overhead, to the side, floor and back up. Keep the head up.

(continued...)

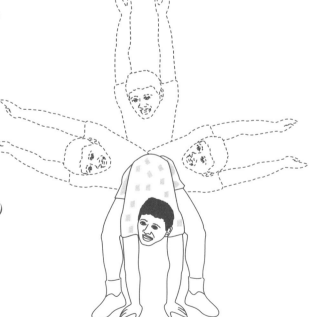

Improving Body Composition and Flexibility

Straddle stretch (for legs and lower back)—Stretch forward with upper body between open legs. Keep knees facing up and legs and back straight. *Note:* For students who are less flexible, placing the hands behind the thighs is a good modification.

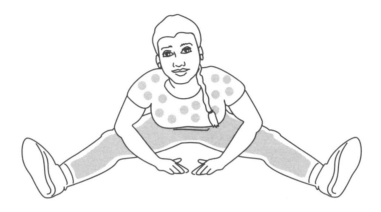

Butterfly stretch (for inner thighs)—Bring heels together and toward the body. Grab ankles and press knees toward the floor. Stretch the torso forward.

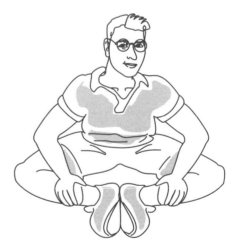

IMPROVING MUSCULAR STRENGTH AND ENDURANCE

Muscular strength and endurance can be improved by demanding more work from one's muscles. This is called *overloading*. This is why it's important not to quit exercising when muscles start to tire.

Muscular training is very specific. To build up the arms, the arm muscles must be overloaded. Overloading the leg muscles will not increase arm strength.

REPS AND SETS

Reps and *sets* are the building blocks of the workout. Reps are repetitions of an exercise. To do a sit-up for 8 reps means to perform it 8 times in a row before resting. A set is 1 group of reps followed by a rest interval. Performing 8 sit-ups, resting 45 seconds to a minute, then doing 8 more sit-ups equals 2 sets.

A workout for muscular strength or endurance should include 5–12 reps of each exercise for 3 sets. When an exercise becomes easy to do, add 2-1/2 to 5 pounds to the barbell, dumbbells or other equipment.

WAYS TO IMPROVE STRENGTH AND ENDURANCE

The following methods are popular ways to improve muscular strength and endurance:
- free weights (hand-held weights, dumbbells and barbells)
- machines (Universal, Hydrofitness, Nautilus, Taurus and Avita)
- calisthenics (sit-ups, push-ups, leg raises, etc.)

Improving muscular strength is different from improving muscular endurance. To increase strength, you do a few repetitions (usually 5–8) with heavy loads. Muscular endurance is developed by doing more repetitions (usually 10–14) with lighter loads.

GUIDELINES FOR SAFELY IMPROVING MUSCULAR STRENGTH AND ENDURANCE
- Have an exercise instructor demonstrate the proper use of any equipment.
- Don't exercise alone. Use a spotter if using barbells.
- Warm up and stretch before beginning.
- Gradually increase the level of exercise.
- Allow at least 48 hours for muscles to recover from a workout. Workouts on consecutive days do more harm than good, because the body cannot adapt that quickly.
- Don't let more than 4 days pass without working out. Muscles will begin to break down if more than 3 or 4 days pass without exercise.
- Exhale during exertion and inhale when releasing.

(continued...)

IMPROVING MUSCULAR STRENGTH AND ENDURANCE

EXERCISES FOR MUSCULAR STRENGTH AND ENDURANCE

The following exercises will improve muscular strength and endurance.

High jumper (for hips and upper and lower legs)—Start with knees slightly bent. Jump as high as possible while raising both arms.

Outer-thigh raise (for outer thigh and hip)—Rest on forearm and hip, with bottom leg bent at a 90-degree angle and top leg raised slightly. Slowly lift and lower top leg in a straight line with body. Repeat with the other leg.

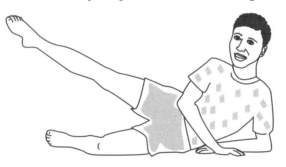

Inner-thigh raise (for inner thighs)—Rest on hip with forearm and bent upper leg helping you balance. Rotate bottom leg out so that heel is turned up and toes are turned down. Keep foot flexed and lift leg as high as possible without rolling hip back. Repeat with the other leg.

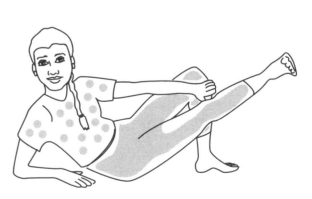

(continued…)

IMPROVING MUSCULAR STRENGTH AND ENDURANCE

Sit-ups (for abdominals)—Lie on back with knees flexed and feet on the floor. Place heels 12 to 18 inches from the buttocks. Cross arms on the chest with hands on opposite shoulders. Tuck chin toward the chest. Tighten abdominal muscles to curl shoulders and upper back off the floor. Keep feet on the floor.

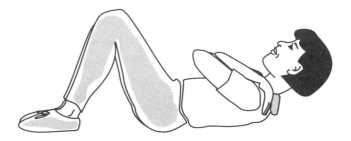

Push-ups (modified) (for chest, shoulders and arms)—Assume a front-leaning position with knees bent up and hands under shoulders. Lower the chest toward the floor. Raise and repeat.

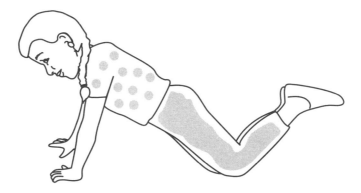

Push-ups (advanced) (for chest, shoulders and arms)—Assume a front-leaning position. Lower the chest toward the floor. Raise and repeat.

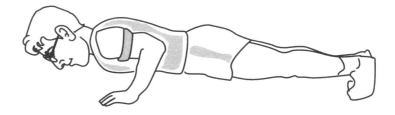

FITNESS FOCUS

KEY

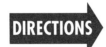 **DIRECTIONS** Read the following case studies. Discuss the case studies with your group and decide which element of fitness each person needs to improve. Then write an exercise prescription for each person. List specific ways in which the element of fitness can be improved.

CLEO

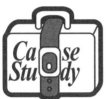 Cleo had been excited about the big Christmas dance for weeks, because Julio had asked her to go with him. The band was great and all her friends were there. The decorations looked terrific, and Julio and Cleo were having a great time.

But after about 30 minutes of nonstop dancing, Cleo had to sit out some of the dances. She couldn't catch her breath. She just didn't seem to have the energy to keep going.

Element of fitness that needs improvement: ***aerobic capacity***

Fitness prescription: ***Warm up by walking briskly for 5 minutes, then stretch for 5–10 minutes. Walk for at least 20 minutes, 3–5 times per week, and gradually increase to a comfortable jog, 3–5 times per week. Cool down by walking for 5 minutes, then stretch 5–10 minutes after each exercise session.***

RAPHAEL

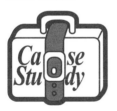 School was almost over, and Raphael was looking forward to some lazy afternoons with friends at the lake. He got his swimsuit from his bottom drawer and pulled it on. Uh oh! The suit seemed to be a little tighter this year. Raphael decided to take a look in the mirror. Oops! He noticed a few bulges and ripples that weren't there last year.

Raphael was concerned about his appearance. In only a couple of months, the lake would be warm enough for swimming.

Element of fitness that needs improvement: ***body composition***

Fitness prescription: ***Increase physical activity, especially aerobic exercise. For example, play basketball for at least 30 minutes after school, 3–5 times per week. Eat a variety of foods, while avoiding fats and sugar. Include lots of fruits, vegetables and whole-grain products.***

(continued...)

NIKKI

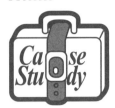

Nikki is pregnant with her first baby. She's very excited. But lately, Nikki has developed a backache that just won't go away. She bent over the other day to pick up a book and had trouble straightening up.

Element of fitness that needs improvement: ***flexibility***

Fitness prescription: ***Perform static stretching every day after warming up. Do 5 neck stretches, 5 shoulder rolls, 5 body circles, 5 straddle stretches and 5 butterfly stretches.***

LEONA

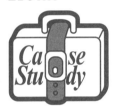

Leona has always helped her neighbors out and earned a little spending money by raking leaves in the fall. This October, Leona discovered that she got tired before she finished raking the first yard. The next day she was so sore she could hardly get out of bed.

Element of fitness that needs improvement: ***muscular endurance***

Fitness prescription: ***Do calisthenics such as sit-ups, push-ups and leg raises. Perform 3 sets, with 10–14 repetitions of each exercise per set.***

MITCH

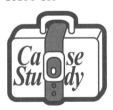

Mitch had been bragging about the used car he bought from his cousin. It had a great sound system and a new paint job. Mitch drove his new car to the Yogurt Factory for a waffle cone. When he was ready to leave, he couldn't get the car started. He tried to push the car while his girlfriend steered, but it wouldn't budge.

Element of fitness that needs improvement: ***muscular strength***

Fitness prescription: ***Join a community health club and use the exercise machines or free weights. Perform 3 sets of 5–8 repetitions. If Mitch can't join a club, he can do calisthenics.***

BE PREPARED

TIME

2 periods

ACTIVITIES

1. The Truth About Fitness
2. Preparing for Fitness
3. Successful Fitness Programs

BE PREPARED

OBJECTIVES

Students will be able to:

1. Identify common myths associated with fitness.

2. Describe factors that influence the success of a fitness program.

GETTING STARTED

Copy for each student:

- An Overheard Conversation (6.1)

Make transparency of:

- Planning for Fitness (6.2)
- Effects of Steroids (6.3)

Copy for one-third of the class:

- Running the 10K (6.4)
- Hiking Pinnacle Mountain (6.5)
- Playing in the Hoopfest (6.6)

UNIT OVERVIEW

Improving or maintaining fitness takes time and perseverance. Many overly enthusiastic exercisers end up on the sidelines because they ignored such factors as equipment, weather or their own bodies' danger signals. In addition, many people fail to recognize the roles of fluid replacement, rest, nutrition and drug use as they relate to fitness. This lesson helps students identify factors that influence the success of a fitness program.

MAIN POINTS

* Appropriate dress can make exercise more enjoyable and reduce the risk of weather-related problems.
* Drinking water is the best way to replace the fluids lost during physical activity.
* A balanced diet provides adequate nutrition for the demands of physical activity.
* Steroid use can damage body organs and cause psychological changes.
* Proper exercise equipment decreases wear and tear on the body and reduces the risk of injury.
* Adequate sleep prepares the body for physical activity and contributes to overall fitness.

REVIEW

To increase your understanding of the factors that influence the success of fitness regimens, review **Fitness Factors** *Instant Expert* (p. 77).

VOCABULARY

steroids—Drugs that function like the male hormone testosterone.

supplements—Vitamins, minerals or proteins that are taken in tablet or capsule form.

1. The Truth About Fitness

40 minutes

MATERIALS

- An Overheard Conversation (6.1)
- transparency of Planning for Fitness (6.2)
- transparency of Effects of Steroids (6.3)

Groups discuss fitness myths

Divide the class into small groups. Distribute the An Overheard Conversation activity sheet and explain the group assignment:

- Read and discuss the conversation on the activity sheet
- Decide whether the highlighted statements are true or false.
- Circle the statements the group thinks are true.

Discuss successful fitness programs

Display the Planning For Fitness transparency. Review each of the factors that contribute to the success of a fitness program, using the Fitness Factors *Instant Expert* as a guide.

(continued...)

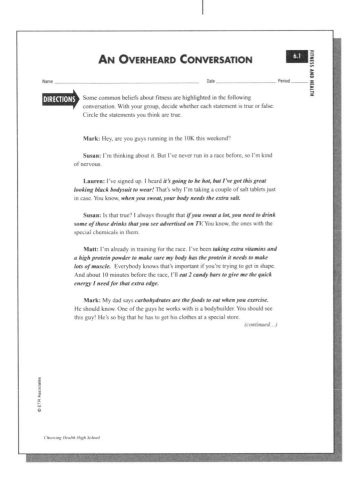

An Overheard Conversation — 6.1 — FITNESS AND HEALTH

Name _____ Date _____ Period _____

DIRECTIONS Some common beliefs about fitness are highlighted in the following conversation. With your group, decide whether each statement is true or false. Circle the statements you think are true.

Mark: Hey, are you guys running in the 10K this weekend?

Susan: I'm thinking about it. But I've never run in a race before, so I'm kind of nervous.

Lauren: I've signed up. I heard *it's going to be hot, but I've got this great looking black bodysuit to wear!* That's why I'm taking a couple of salt tablets just in case. You know, *when you sweat, your body needs the extra salt.*

Susan: Is that true? I always thought that *if you sweat a lot, you need to drink some of those drinks that you see advertised on TV.* You know, the ones with the special chemicals in them.

Matt: I'm already in training for the race. I've been *taking extra vitamins and a high protein powder to make sure my body has the protein it needs to make lots of muscle.* Everybody knows that's important if you're trying to get in shape. And about 10 minutes before the race, I'll *eat 2 candy bars to give me the quick energy I need for that extra edge.*

Mark: My dad says *carbohydrates are the foods to eat when you exercise.* He should know. One of the guys he works with is a bodybuilder. You should see this guy! He's so big that he has to get his clothes at a special store.

(continued...)

© ETR Associates

Choosing Health High School

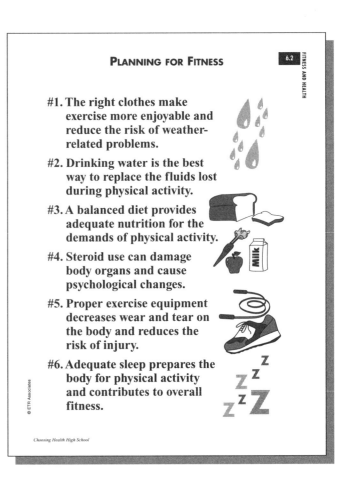

Planning for Fitness — 6.2 — FITNESS AND HEALTH

#1. The right clothes make exercise more enjoyable and reduce the risk of weather-related problems.

#2. Drinking water is the best way to replace the fluids lost during physical activity.

#3. A balanced diet provides adequate nutrition for the demands of physical activity.

#4. Steroid use can damage body organs and cause psychological changes.

#5. Proper exercise equipment decreases wear and tear on the body and reduces the risk of injury.

#6. Adequate sleep prepares the body for physical activity and contributes to overall fitness.

© ETR Associates

Choosing Health High School

1. THE TRUTH ABOUT FITNESS

CONTINUED

Discuss steroids

Display the **Effects of Steroids** transparency. Emphasize the health risks associated with the use of these drugs, using the **Fitness Factors** *Instant Expert* as a guide.

Discuss fitness myths

Ask students to look again at the **An Overheard Conversation** activity sheet. Would any of their answers change based on the class discussion?

Ongoing Assessment Look for students' ability to differentiate valid statements about exercise from those statements that are myths. See the **An Overheard Conversation** *Key* for specific criteria.

EXTEND THE LEARNING

Have students recall other "facts/myths" they've heard about exercise, research these "facts" and then report their findings to the class.

✳

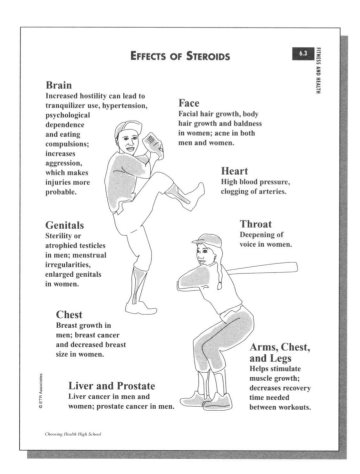

EFFECTS OF STEROIDS

FITNESS AND HEALTH

Brain
Increased hostility can lead to tranquilizer use, hypertension, psychological dependence and eating compulsions; increases aggression, which makes injuries more probable.

Face
Facial hair growth, body hair growth and baldness in women; acne in both men and women.

Heart
High blood pressure, clogging of arteries.

Genitals
Sterility or atrophied testicles in men; menstrual irregularities, enlarged genitals in women.

Throat
Deepening of voice in women.

Chest
Breast growth in men; breast cancer and decreased breast size in women.

Arms, Chest, and Legs
Helps stimulate muscle growth; decreases recovery time needed between workouts.

Liver and Prostate
Liver cancer in men and women; prostate cancer in men.

© ETR Associates

Choosing Health High School

2. PREPARING FOR FITNESS

25 minutes

MATERIALS

- Running the 10K (6.4)
- Hiking Pinnacle Mountain (6.5)
- Playing in the Hoopfest (6.6)

Groups suggest fitness preparations

Have students return to their small groups from Activity 1. Allow groups to select 1 of the activity sheets—**Running the 10K, Hiking Pinnacle Mountain** or **Playing in the Hoopfest**. Explain the group assignment:

- Choose a reader to read the situation and a reporter to report group answers to the class.
- Discuss the situation.
- Agree on a group answer to the questions.

Groups report

Have a reporter from each group report the group's answers to the class. As reports are made, confirm the appropriateness of correct responses and correct any misinformation.

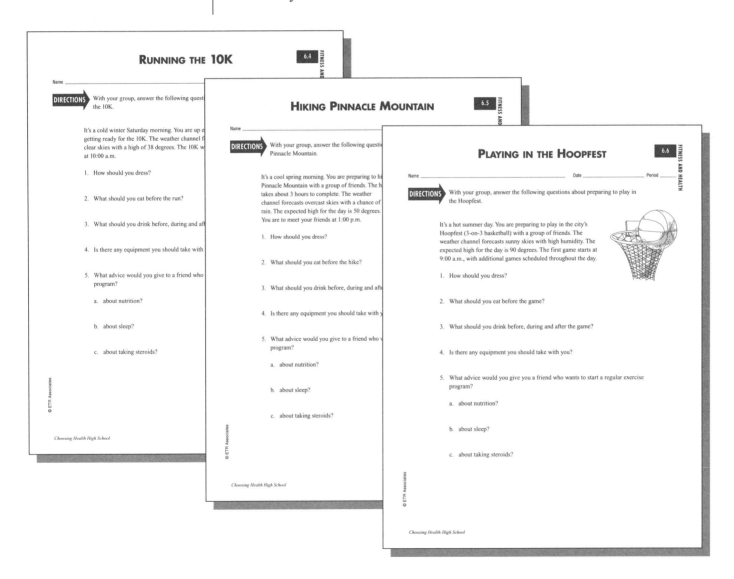

3. SUCCESSFUL FITNESS PROGRAMS

Groups discuss fitness interviews

Divide students into small groups to review and report on the interviews they conducted in Unit 1. They will be applying their new knowledge (from Unit 6) to the information gained from the interviewing activity.

Ask groups to share interesting information from their interview reports. They should look at the fitness plans interviewees described and discuss:

- benefits of exercises (walking, bicycling, weight lifting, etc.)
- the elements of fitness the exercises improve (aerobic capacity, flexibility, muscular strength and endurance, body composition)
- fluid replacement, eating habits and sleep habits (Do they meet guidelines discussed in class?)
- advice to beginning exercisers
- factors that contribute to the success of an exercise program

Groups report

Ask each group to summarize for the class. As groups report, compile a class list of the factors that contribute to a successful exercise program.

25 minutes

MATERIALS

- Fitness Interview (1.7), from Unit 1, Activity 5

COMMUNITY LINK

Have students interview persons involved in a variety of exercise activities (for example, racquetball, rapelling, mountain biking). Ask students to determine the type of equipment needed for the activity.

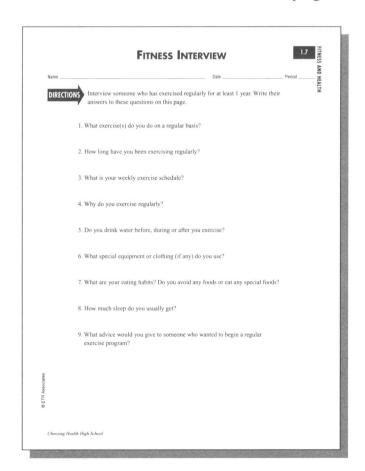

FITNESS INTERVIEW   1.7

Name _____ Date _____ Period _____

DIRECTIONS ▶ Interview someone who has exercised regularly for at least 1 year. Write their answers to these questions on this page.

1. What exercise(s) do you do on a regular basis?

2. How long have you been exercising regularly?

3. What is your weekly exercise schedule?

4. Why do you exercise regularly?

5. Do you drink water before, during or after you exercise?

6. What special equipment or clothing (if any) do you use?

7. What are your eating habits? Do you avoid any foods or eat any special foods?

8. How much sleep do you usually get?

9. What advice would you give to someone who wanted to begin a regular exercise program?

© ETR Associates

Choosing Health High School

EVALUATION

10 minutes

REVIEW

♦ An Overheard Conversation *Key* (p. 80)

MATERIALS

♦ completed An Overheard Conversation, from Activity 1

OBJECTIVE 1

Students will be able to:

> **Identify common myths associated with fitness.**

Allow students to redo the **An Overheard Conversation** activity sheet based on what they learned in this unit. Compare these answers to the first to assess their ability to identify fitness myths.

CRITERIA

See the **An Overheard Conversation** *Key* for evaluation criteria.

OBJECTIVE 2

Students will be able to:

> **Describe factors that influence the success of a fitness program.**

Observe student work in small groups and group reports for their knowledge of factors that influence the success of a fitness program.

CRITERIA

Assess students' ability to describe factors that positively influence the success of a fitness program. Factors should include:

- appropriate dress for the activity and weather
- proper fluid replacement (water)
- adequate equipment for the activity
- a balanced diet
- adequate sleep
- avoidance of steroids

FITNESS FACTORS

Many factors influence the success of fitness programs. Important considerations include:

- weather
- fluid replacement
- nutrition
- equipment
- rest

Unfortunately, some people are tempted to use drugs to improve their performance. Students must be alerted to the dangers of such drug use.

PREPARING FOR WEATHER

When planning to exercise, consider the weather (temperature and humidity) and dress accordingly. In hot weather, light colors and fabrics allow the body to dissipate the heat. Never wear rubberized or plastic clothing. Take it easy during the first few hot days to allow your body to get used to warmer weather. Before you feel weak and tired, stop and drink several ounces of water.

Protect yourself from cold weather by covering as much of your body as possible. Dress in layers of clothing that you can remove as you begin to warm up. Choose dark colors that absorb heat.

About 40 percent of body heat is lost through the head and neck, so wear a cap or other head covering. The areas most sensitive to cold are fingers, toes and ears. Protecting these with mittens, wool socks and caps reduces the discomfort and dangers of exposure to low temperatures.

REPLACING FLUIDS

The body loses fluid through sweating even in cool temperatures. Unfortunately, thirst is not always a good indicator of the body's need for fluid during physical activity. Therefore, people should make a conscious effort to drink enough fluids when exercising.

Plain water is the ideal fluid replacement. Consuming sugary drinks (soft drinks) prior to exercising can decrease endurance, due to the body's production of insulin in response to the sugar.

Beverages containing caffeine (colas, teas and coffee) should also be avoided, because they may stimulate fluid loss in the body. Alcohol hampers coordination and impairs performance, due to the depressant effect of the drug. In addition, alcohol promotes the loss of fluid from the body.

(continued...)

FITNESS FACTORS

Americans take in more than enough salt through the foods they eat to replace salt lost in sweating. Never take salt tablets. They can lead to dehydration and elevate blood pressure.

SUPPLYING NUTRIENTS

For most people who exercise to improve fitness, eating a balanced diet is all that is required to supply the body with the necessary nutrients. In some endurance sports such as running marathons, athletes engage in complex *carbohydrate(hydrate) loading* to increase the energy sources (glycogen) in their muscles.

But for less strenuous levels of physical activity, the body's fuel comes from foods eaten hours, even days, earlier. For this reason, eating a candy bar or other food high in sugar before exercising will not provide the sustained energy needed.

Supplements (vitamins, minerals and protein powders) are unnecessary for active people who eat a balanced diet. Excessive amounts of vitamins and minerals can be dangerous and do not provide the combination of nutrients that are supplied by eating a variety of foods.

SELECTING EQUIPMENT

Proper equipment makes a big difference in how well you perform and your enjoyment of the activity. Good shoes are essential for almost all sports and activities. Boots are important for hiking or skiing. Appropriate footwear is necessary for aerobic dance and all running sports. A proper fit is important, too. The proper shoes not only protect the body from wear and tear, but minimize the risk of injury.

Other activities may require specialized equipment, such as gloves, goggles, rackets, eye protectors, bicycles and specialized clothing. If participants usually wear or use certain items, there must be a valid reason.

Selecting equipment can be confusing because of the variations in design and price. Some equipment may be barely adequate. Before purchasing, observe what others are using and ask experienced participants for advice. If still in doubt, consider renting first and buying later.

REST

Sleep is an indispensable part of a fitness program. During sleep, we recover from physical and emotional stresses and injuries. The amount of sleep needed varies from one individual to the next. In fact, for each individual, sleep needs vary according to one's activity level, overall health and age.

(continued...)

FITNESS FACTORS

Young people generally require about 8 hours of sleep per night. We know that growth hormone is secreted almost exclusively during sleep—and growth hormone provides for the growth and repair of body cells.

When we fail to get enough sleep, all body systems work less efficiently. We become irritable, have trouble concentrating and lose coordination. People who go without sleep too long may have hallucinations.

USING STEROIDS

Anabolic steroids are drugs that function like the male hormone testosterone. Steroids can be taken in tablet form or by injection. Steroids are used medically to treat certain diseases and people who have growth disorders. Bodybuilders and other athletes may use steroids in an effort to stimulate muscle growth and weight gain. Steroids also increase aggression, which may make the athlete train harder.

Steroids promote increased strength and bulk; however, experts agree the health risks outweigh any benefits. Some possible effects include liver damage, hypertension, certain forms of cancer, heart disease, muscle cramps, acne and gastrointestinal distress.

Men who take steroids may experience breast growth, reduced sperm production and shrinking of the testicles. Side effects for women include growth of facial and body hair, baldness, a lowering of the voice, decreased breast size, menstrual irregularities and enlarged genitals.

AN OVERHEARD CONVERSATION

KEY

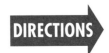 Some common beliefs about fitness are highlighted in the following conversation. With your group, decide whether each statement is true or false. Circle the statements you think are true.

Mark: Hey, are you guys running in the 10K this weekend?

Susan: I'm thinking about it. But I've never run in a race before, so I'm kind of nervous.

Lauren: I've signed up. I heard *it's going to be hot, but I've got this great looking black bodysuit to wear!* ***(False: See "Planning for Fitness" #1.)*** That's why I'm taking a couple of salt tablets just in case. You know, *when you sweat, your body needs the extra salt.* ***(False: See "Planning for Fitness" #2.)***

Susan: Is that true? I always thought that *if you sweat a lot, you need to drink some of those drinks that you see advertised on TV.* You know, the ones with the special chemicals in them. ***(False: See "Planning for Fitness" #2.)***

Matt: I'm already in training for the race. I've been *taking extra vitamins and a high protein powder to make sure my body has the protein it needs to make lots of muscle.* ***(False: See "Planning for Fitness" #3.)*** Everybody knows that's important if you're trying to get in shape. And about 10 minutes before the race, I'll *eat 2 candy bars to give me the quick energy I need for that extra edge.* ***(False: See "Planning for Fitness" #3.)***

Mark: My dad says *carbohydrates are the foods to eat when you exercise.* ***(False: See "Planning for Fitness" #3.)*** He should know. One of the guys he works with is a bodybuilder. You should see this guy! He's so big that he has to get his clothes at a special store.

(continued...)

KEY, CONTINUED

Lauren: I'll bet your dad's friend takes steroids. I've heard *steroids are really dangerous. (True: See "Planning for Fitness" #4.)* I read in the newspaper about a man who grew breasts after he took steroids and a teenager who got a liver disease!

Matt: I don't believe that garbage. *Steroids only make your muscles grow faster and stronger. (False: See "Planning for Fitness" #4.)* No one would take them if they did weird things to your body.

Susan: Who knows about that stuff? I'd like to go with you guys, but I don't have any running shoes.

Mark: Just wear those shoes you have on. *Your shoes really don't matter. (False: See "Planning for Fitness" #5.)* You're not running the Boston Marathon.

Susan: I've got to go. See you guys this weekend. Be sure to get rested up for the 10K. You know, *you need 2–3 extra hours of sleep when you're a high-powered athlete. (False: See "Planning for Fitness" #6.)*

UNIT

7

PUTTING IT ALL TOGETHER

TIME
1–2 periods

ACTIVITIES
1. What Are Your Goals?
2. What Are Your Plans?
3. How Did You Do?

PUTTING IT ALL TOGETHER

OBJECTIVES

Students will be able to:

1. Identify personal goals for fitness.

2. Develop a personal exercise plan.

GETTING STARTED

Copy for each student:

- Setting Fitness Goals (7.1)
- Developing Your Fitness Plan (7.3)
- Fitness Plan (7.5)
- Fitness Record (7.7)

Make transparency of:

- Ratings for Popular Activities (7.2)
- Developing Your Fitness Plan Example (7.4)
- Fitness Plan Example (7.6)

UNIT OVERVIEW

PURPOSE

There is a close relationship between physical fitness and overall lifestyle. Fitness has an impact on attitude, eating and sleeping habits and body awareness. This lesson deals with the mental attitude and lifestyle that are linked to succeeding at beginning and maintaining regular exercise.

MAIN POINTS

✸ Goal setting is an important part of developing personal fitness.

✸ Developing a personal fitness plan can improve chances of success in establishing a long-term fitness program.

REVIEW

To increase your understanding of the steps for setting fitness goals, review **Planning for Fitness** *Instant Expert* (p. 92).

VOCABULARY

goal—An end that a person aims to reach or accomplish.

habit—An act that is done often, in a certain way, and has become automatic.

plan—A scheme for making, doing or arranging something; a program; a schedule.

1. WHAT ARE YOUR GOALS?

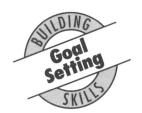

10 minutes

MATERIALS

◆ Setting Fitness Goals (7.1)

FAMILY LINK

Have students interview family members about goals they achieved and how they achieved them.

During a follow-up discussion, emphasize that accomplishing a goal usually takes time, planning and effort.

Students determine goals

Distribute the **Setting Fitness Goals** activity sheet and have students complete it to determine their motivations for fitness.

Discuss goal setting

Conduct a brief class discussion about goal setting. Ask students:

- Why do people set goals?
- How can we improve our chances of reaching a goal?

Review the following steps that can help people reach their goals:

- Make the goal realistic.
- Get friends and family to support you emotionally.
- Write the goal down and put it where you can see it.
- Develop a plan.
- Outline step-by-step how to reach your goal.

Ongoing Assessment Look for students' understanding that people set goals to order and gain control of their lives and get what they want. Students should be able to identify specific steps that will work for them.

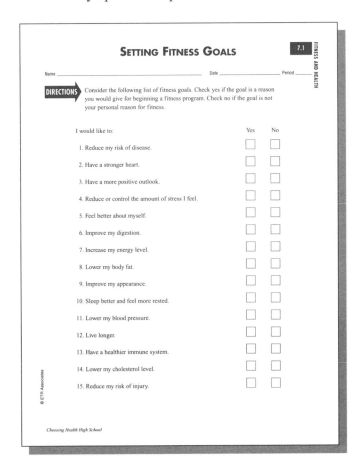

2. WHAT ARE YOUR PLANS?

Brainstorm fitness activities

Conduct a brainstorming session to identify a variety of fitness activities. List responses on the board.

Discuss fitness activities

Discuss the different elements of fitness addressed by the activities students brainstormed. Display the **Ratings for Popular Activities** transparency to help students identify the various elements addressed by different activities. Ask students:

- What activities do you enjoy?
- What elements of fitness do these activities address?

(continued...)

35 minutes

MATERIALS

- transparency of Ratings for Popular Activities (7.2)
- Developing Your Fitness Plan (7.3)
- transparency of Developing Your Fitness Plan Example (7.4)
- Fitness Plan (7.5)
- transparency of Fitness Plan Example (7.6)

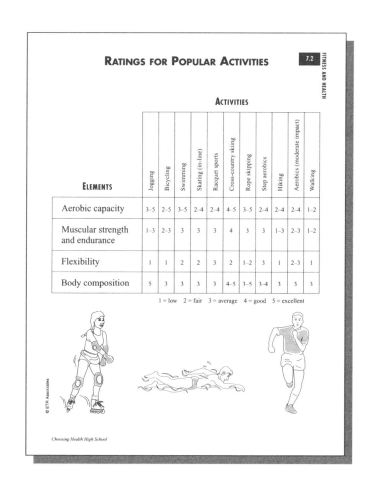

RATINGS FOR POPULAR ACTIVITIES | 7.2

ACTIVITIES

ELEMENTS	Jogging	Bicycling	Swimming	Skating (in-line)	Racquet sports	Cross-country skiing	Rope skipping	Step aerobics	Hiking	Aerobics (moderate impact)	Walking
Aerobic capacity	3–5	2–5	3–5	2–4	2–4	4–5	3–5	2–4	2–4	2–4	1–2
Muscular strength and endurance	1–3	2–3	3	3	3	4	3	3	1–3	2–3	1–2
Flexibility	1	1	2	2	3	2	1–2	3	1	2–3	1
Body composition	5	3	3	3	3	4–5	3–5	3-4	3	3	3

1 = low   2 = fair   3 = average   4 = good   5 = excellent

© ETR Associates

Choosing Health High School

2. WHAT ARE YOUR PLANS?

MEETING STUDENT NEEDS

Help students be realistic in developing their plans. Some students may already be very active and engage in regular exercise. Others may be less active and will benefit from simply walking several times each week. Encourage the more sedentary students to begin slowly and support small changes in their activity levels.

Students develop fitness plans

Distribute the **Developing Your Fitness Plan** activity sheet. Explain that developing a plan helps people reach their goals.

Display the **Developing Your Fitness Plan Example** transparency as you discuss the steps of the process. After discussing each step, ask students to complete that section of the activity sheet.

- *Step 1—Make it personal.* Refer to the Assess Your Fitness activity sheet completed in Unit 2. Look at the elements you most need to improve and try to incorporate as many elements as possible into your fitness program.
- *Step 2—Motivate yourself.* Motivation is a common barrier to fitness. Remind yourself of your fitness goals (see Activity 1). Make exercise enjoyable by choosing activities you like. Support from family members and friends can also help you maintain your enthusiasm for exercise.

(continued...)

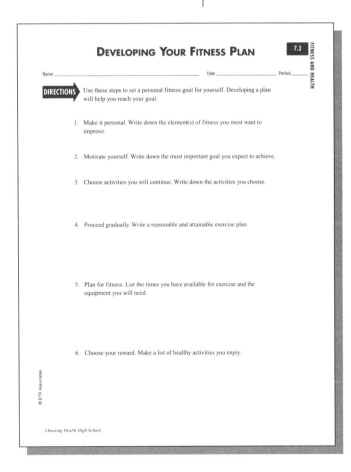

DEVELOPING YOUR FITNESS PLAN   7.3   FITNESS AND HEALTH

Name _____ Date _____ Period _____

DIRECTIONS Use these steps to set a personal fitness goal for yourself. Developing a plan will help you reach your goal.

1. Make it personal. Write down the element(s) of fitness you most want to improve.

2. Motivate yourself. Write down the most important goal you expect to achieve.

3. Choose activities you will continue. Write down the activities you choose.

4. Proceed gradually. Write a reasonable and attainable exercise plan.

5. Plan for fitness. List the times you have available for exercise and the equipment you will need.

6. Choose your reward. Make a list of healthy activities you enjoy.

© ETR Associates

Choosing Health High School

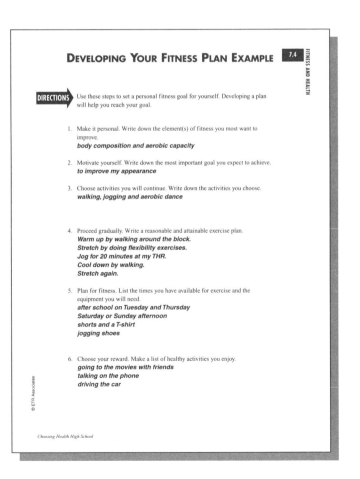

DEVELOPING YOUR FITNESS PLAN EXAMPLE   7.4   FITNESS AND HEALTH

DIRECTIONS Use these steps to set a personal fitness goal for yourself. Developing a plan will help you reach your goal.

1. Make it personal. Write down the element(s) of fitness you most want to improve.
   body composition and aerobic capacity

2. Motivate yourself. Write down the most important goal you expect to achieve.
   to improve my appearance

3. Choose activities you will continue. Write down the activities you choose.
   walking, jogging and aerobic dance

4. Proceed gradually. Write a reasonable and attainable exercise plan.
   Warm up by walking around the block.
   Stretch by doing flexibility exercises.
   Jog for 20 minutes at my THR.
   Cool down by walking.
   Stretch again.

5. Plan for fitness. List the times you have available for exercise and the equipment you will need.
   after school on Tuesday and Thursday
   Saturday or Sunday afternoon
   shorts and a T-shirt
   jogging shoes

6. Choose your reward. Make a list of healthy activities you enjoy.
   going to the movies with friends
   talking on the phone
   driving the car

© ETR Associates

Choosing Health High School

2. WHAT ARE YOUR PLANS?

CONTINUED

- **Step 3—Choose activities you will continue.** Think about the activities that are convenient and that you will enjoy. Choose something you like to do. Consider your interests and skills as well as social factors when you select an activity.
- **Step 4—Proceed gradually.** Even though you may want to progress quickly, you must give your body a chance to adjust, especially if you have not exercised in a while. It is important to set reasonable and attainable goals for yourself.
- **Step 5—Plan for fitness.** The barrier to fitness that people cite most often is a lack of time. Often, people fail to exercise because they think it will take a lot of time. However, planning the time for exercise into your weekly schedule is just like making plans for any other worthwhile activity.
- **Step 6—Choose your reward.** Think of healthy ways to reward yourself, and follow through when you follow your exercise plan. Rewards can be physical, emotional or social.

EXTEND THE LEARNING

Ask volunteers to share goals they have set for themselves and how they plan to achieve them.

Students plan fitness activities

Distribute the **Fitness Plan** activity sheet. Use the **Fitness Plan Example** transparency to illustrate how to fill in the chart. Have students fill in a plan for exercise for the next week.

FITNESS PLAN `7.5` FITNESS AND HEALTH

Name _____ Date _____ Period _____

Week of: _____

Goal for the week:

Day	Activity	Time	Equipment	Reward
Sunday				
Monday				
Tuesday				
Wednesday				
Thursday				
Friday				
Saturday				

© ETR Associates

Choosing Health High School

FITNESS PLAN EXAMPLE `7.6` FITNESS AND HEALTH

Week of: _April 22–28_

Goal for the week:
Increase amount of jogging time to 25 minutes.
Spend 5 minutes stretching after jogging.

Day	Activity	Time	Equipment	Reward
Sunday	Walk to Carrie's	afternoon	comfortable shoes	talk to Carrie
Monday	Stretch—warm-up—jog 25 minutes—cool down—stretch	afternoon	jogging shoes, shorts and shirt	hot shower
Tuesday	none	none	none	—
Wednesday	Stretch—warm-up—bicycle—cool down—stretch	4 p.m.	bicycle and shorts	listen to music
Thursday	walk to and from school	morning & afternoon	none	rent a video
Friday	stretch—warm-up—jog 25 minutes—cool down—stretch	after school	jogging shoes, shorts and shirt	proud feeling of accomplishment
Saturday	Basketball	afternoon	tennis shoes and shorts	hang out with friends

© ETR Associates

Choosing Health High School

---

3. HOW DID YOU DO?

15 minutes

A SELF-ASSESSMENT ACTIVITY

MATERIALS

◆ Fitness Record (7.7)

MEETING STUDENT NEEDS

Acknowledge that working on the body takes determination. Remind students not to expect miracles in a week, but to view the week as a beginning if they have not had a regular exercise program. Students who exercise regularly may use the activity sheet as a checkup.

EXTEND THE LEARNING

You may want to extend this assignment by having students complete additional Fitness Record activity sheets periodically over the semester or school year.

Students monitor progress

Distribute the **Fitness Record** activity sheet. Point out that it has the same elements as the **Fitness Plan**. This will allow them to see how well they were able to plan. Ask students to keep a record of their fitness activities for 1 week.

Evaluate plans

At the end of the week, students should compare plans with actual accomplishments recorded on the **Fitness Record**. Ask students to readjust plans based on actual exercise. Point out that the readjustment step is an ongoing part of goal setting and planning.

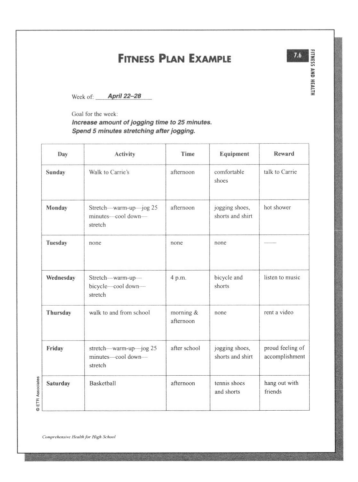

FITNESS PLAN EXAMPLE   7.6

Week of: _____April 22–28_____

Goal for the week:
Increase amount of jogging time to 25 minutes.
Spend 5 minutes stretching after jogging.

Day	Activity	Time	Equipment	Reward
Sunday	Walk to Carrie's	afternoon	comfortable shoes	talk to Carrie
Monday	Stretch—warm-up—jog 25 minutes—cool down—stretch	afternoon	jogging shoes, shorts and shirt	hot shower
Tuesday	none	none	none	—
Wednesday	Stretch—warm-up—bicycle—cool down—stretch	4 p.m.	bicycle and shorts	listen to music
Thursday	walk to and from school	morning & afternoon	none	rent a video
Friday	stretch—warm-up—jog 25 minutes—cool down—stretch	after school	jogging shoes, shorts and shirt	proud feeling of accomplishment
Saturday	Basketball	afternoon	tennis shoes and shorts	hang out with friends

© ETR Associates

Comprehensive Health for High School

EVALUATION

OBJECTIVE 1

Students will be able to:

Identify personal goals for fitness.

Review students' work on the **Setting Fitness Goals** activity sheet.

CRITERIA

Look for students to identify personal reasons to achieve fitness.

MATERIALS

♦ completed Setting Fitness Goals (7.1), from Activity 1

OBJECTIVE 2

Students will be able to:

Develop a personal exercise plan.

Review students' work on the **Developing Your Fitness Plan** and **Fitness Plan** activity sheets to assess their ability to develop an exercise plan.

CRITERIA

Look for:

- personalized goals
- activities that match the student's interests and abilities
- realistic times for exercise
- healthy rewards

MATERIALS

♦ completed Developing Your Fitness Plan (7.3), from Activity 2
♦ completed Fitness Plan (7.5), from Activity 2

PLANNING FOR FITNESS

Getting ready for exercise means being psychologically ready, as well as selecting the appropriate activities and having the proper equipment. All of these factors influence success in starting or maintaining a fitness program. Setting goals for fitness helps provide motivation.

SETTING GOALS FOR FITNESS

The following steps are important components of setting fitness goals.

Step 1—Make it personal. A fitness plan should address the areas where improvement is most needed and incorporate as many elements of fitness as possible. These elements can often be combined in a workout. For example, flexibility can be improved by stretching and cooling down as part of an aerobic workout. Calisthenics to improve muscular strength and endurance can also be done as part of a warm-up for an aerobic workout. An aerobic workout will not only improve aerobic capacity but will contribute to healthy body composition as well.

Step 2—Motivate yourself. Motivation is a common barrier to fitness. Choosing activities you like helps make exercise enjoyable. People who are competitive may enjoy racquetball or basketball. People who enjoy being alone may want to choose jogging or swimming. People who like to combine social activity with physical activity could choose walking with a friend. Support from family members and friends also helps maintain enthusiasm for exercise.

Step 3—Choose activities you will continue. Activities should be convenient and enjoyable. Interests and skills, as well as social factors, should be considered. Talking to people who exercise about their experience with certain activities may help people make choices.

A variety of activities may be included. Most people are more likely to continue a fitness program when they have different ways to exercise. Activities to improve aerobic capacity should be included at least 3 days a week—aerobic exercise offers the most health benefits.

Step 4—Proceed gradually. Even though people desire quick progress, the body must be given a chance to adjust, especially for people who have not exercised in a while. Fitness goals should be reasonable and attainable.

New exercisers need to begin gradually and progress at a pace that is comfortable. Listen to the body. People who are just beginning to exercise can expect some soreness; however, extreme or painful soreness probably indicates an effort to progress too rapidly.

(continued...)

PLANNING FOR FITNESS

Step 5—Plan for fitness. The barrier to fitness that people cite most often is a lack of time. Often, people fail to exercise because they think it means taking a lot of time. However, planning the time for exercise into a weekly schedule is just like making plans for any other worthwhile activity. Planning for fitness also means having the appropriate equipment available and in good repair.

Step 6—Choose your reward. Think of healthy ways to reward yourself, and follow through when you follow your exercise plan. Rewards can be physical, emotional or social. For example: Spending time with a friend or calling someone on the telephone is a social reward. Taking a bubble bath or taking a nap is a physical reward. Emotional rewards may include doing something special or simply acknowledging accomplishments.

FINAL
EVALUATION

FINAL EVALUATION

Evaluate the effectiveness of personal fitness plans

Have students compare their **Fitness Record** with their **Fitness Plan**. Ask them to note places where their actual activities differed from their plans and to answer the following questions on the back of the sheet:

- Was your plan realistic? Why or why not?
- How could your plan be changed to make it more realistic?

Adjust plans and monitor progress

An ongoing fitness regimen needs to be monitored and adjusted regularly to be effective. Help students establish fitness partners to assess fitness plans, monitor progress and provide support over a several month period.

CRITERIA

Look for students to identify similarities and differences between the **Fitness Plan** and **Fitness Record** and to propose ways to make their **Fitness Plan** more realistic. Assess students' fitness partnerships for their success in providing positive support and constructive suggestions for modifications over time. Look for students' ability to stick with a plan.

10 minutes

MATERIALS

- completed Fitness Plan (7.5), from Unit 7, Activity 2
- completed Fitness Record (7.7), from Unit 7, Activity 3

APPENDIXES

Why Comprehensive School Health?

Components of a
Comprehensive Health Program

The Teacher's Role

Teaching Strategies

Glossary

References

WHY COMPREHENSIVE SCHOOL HEALTH?

The quality of life we ultimately achieve is determined in large part by the health decisions we make, the subsequent behaviors we adopt, and the public policies that promote and support the establishment of healthy behaviors.

A healthy student is capable of growing and learning; of producing new knowledge and ideas; of sharing, interacting and living peacefully with others in a complex and changing society. Fostering healthy children is the shared responsibility of families, communities and schools.

Health behaviors, the most important predictors of current and future health status, are influenced by a variety of factors. Factors that lead to and support the establishment of healthy behaviors include:

- awareness and knowledge of health issues
- the skills necessary to practice healthy behaviors
- opportunities to practice healthy behaviors
- support and reinforcement for the practice of healthy behaviors

The perception that a particular healthy behavior is worthwhile often results in young people becoming advocates, encouraging others to adopt the healthy behavior. When these young advocates exert pressure on peers to adopt healthy behaviors, a healthy social norm is established (e.g., tobacco use is unacceptable in this school).

Because health behaviors are learned, they can be shaped and changed. Partnerships between family members, community leaders, teachers and school leaders are a vital key to the initial development and maintenance of children's healthy behaviors and can also play a role in the modification of unhealthy behaviors. Schools, perhaps more than any other single agency in our society, have the opportunity to influence factors that shape the future health and productivity of Americans.

When young people receive reinforcement for the practice of a healthy behavior, they feel good about the healthy behavior. Reinforcement and the subsequent good feeling increase the likelihood that an individual will continue to practice a behavior and thereby establish a positive health habit. The good feeling and the experience of success motivate young people to place a high value on the behavior (e.g., being a nonsmoker is good).

From *Step by Step to Comprehensive School Health,* W. M. Kane (Santa Cruz, CA: ETR Associates, 1992).

COMPONENTS OF A COMPREHENSIVE HEALTH PROGRAM

The school's role in fostering the development of healthy students involves more than providing classes in health. There are 8 components of a comprehensive health education program:

- **School Health Instruction**—Instruction is the in-class aspect of the program. As in other subject areas, a scope of content defines the field. Application of classroom instruction to real life situations is critical.

- **Healthy School Environment**—The school environment includes both the physical and psychological surroundings of students, faculty and staff. The physical environment should be free of hazards; the psychological environment should foster healthy development.

- **School Health Services**—School health services offer a variety of activities that address the health status of students and staff.

- **Physical Education and Fitness**—Participation in physical education and fitness activities promotes healthy development. Students need information about how and why to be active and encouragement to develop skills that will contribute to fitness throughout their lives.

- **School Nutrition and Food Services**—The school's nutritional program provides an excellent opportunity to model healthy behaviors. Schools that provide healthy food choices and discourage availability of unhealthy foods send a clear message to students about the importance of good nutrition.

- **School-Based Counseling and Personal Support**—School counseling and support services play an important role in responding to special needs and providing personal support for individual students, teachers and staff. These services can also provide programs that promote schoolwide mental, emotional and social well-being.

- **Schoolsite Health Promotion**—Health promotion is a combination of educational, organizational and environmental activities designed to encourage students and staff to adopt healthier lifestyles and become better consumers of health care services. It views the school and its activities as a total environment.

- **School, Family and Community Health Promotion Partnerships**—Partnerships that unite schools, families and communities can address communitywide issues. These collaborative partnerships are the cornerstone of health promotion and disease prevention.

The Teacher's Role

The teacher plays a critical role in meeting the challenge to empower students with the knowledge, skills and ability to make healthy behavior choices throughout their lives.

Instruction

Teachers need to provide students with learning opportunities that go beyond knowledge. Instruction must include the chance to practice skills that will help students make healthy decisions.

Involve Families and Communities

The issues in health are real-life issues, issues that families and communities deal with daily. Students need to see the relationship of what they learn at school to what occurs in their homes and their communities.

Model Healthy Behavior

Teachers educate students by their actions too. Students watch the way teachers manage health issues in their own lives. Teachers need to ask themselves if they are modeling the health behaviors they want students to adopt.

Maintain a Healthy Environment

The classroom environment has both physical and emotional aspects. It is the teacher's role to maintain a safe physical environment. It is also critical to provide an environment that is sensitive, respectful and developmentally appropriate.

Establish Groundrules

It is very important to establish classroom groundrules before discussing sensitive topics or issues. Setting and consistently enforcing groundrules establishes an atmosphere of respect, in which students can share and explore their personal thoughts, feelings, opinions and values.

Refer Students to Appropriate Services

Teachers may be the first to notice illness, learning disorders or emotional distress in students. The role of the teacher is one of referral. Most districts have guidelines for teachers to follow.

Legal Compliance

Teachers must make every effort to communicate to parents and other family members about the nature of the curriculum. Instruction about certain topics, such as sexuality, HIV or drug use, often must follow notification guidelines regulated by state law. Most states also require teachers to report any suspected cases of child abuse or neglect.

TEACHING STRATEGIES

The resource books incorporate a variety of instructional strategies. This variety is essential in addressing the needs of different kinds of learners. Different strategies are grouped according to their general education purpose. When sequenced, these strategies are designed to help students acquire the knowledge and skills they need to choose healthy behavior. Strategies are identified with each activity. Some strategies are traditional, while others are more interactive, encouraging students to help each other learn.

The strategies are divided into 4 categories according to their general purpose:

- providing key information
- encouraging creative expression
- sharing thoughts, feelings and opinions
- developing critical thinking

The following list details strategies in each category.

Providing Key Information

Information provides the foundation for learning. Before students can move to higher-level thinking, they need to have information about a topic. In lieu of a textbook, this series uses a variety of strategies to provide students the information they need to take actions for their health.

Anonymous Question Box

An anonymous question box provides the opportunity for all students to get answers to questions they might be hesitant to ask in class. It also gives teachers time to think about answers to difficult questions or to look for more information.

Questions should be reviewed and responded to regularly, and all questions placed in the box should be taken seriously. If you don't know the answer to a question, research it and report back to students.

You may feel that some questions would be better answered privately. Offer students the option of signing their questions if they want a private, written answer. Any questions not answered in class can then be answered privately.

Current Events

Analyzing local, state, national and international current events helps students relate classroom discussion to everyday life. It also helps students understand how local, national and global events and policies affect health status. Resources for current

TEACHING STRATEGIES

events include newspapers, magazines and other periodicals, radio and television programs and news.

Demonstrations and Experiments

Teachers, guest speakers or students can use demonstrations and experiments to show how something works or why something is important. These activities also provide a way to show the correct process for doing something, such as a first-aid procedure.

Demonstrations and experiments should be carefully planned and conducted. They often involve the use of supporting materials.

Games and Puzzles

Games and puzzles can be used to provide a different environment in which learning can take place. They are frequently amusing and sometimes competitive.

Many types of games and puzzles can be adapted to present and review health concepts. It may be a simple question-and-answer game or an adaptation of games such as Bingo, Concentration or Jeopardy. Puzzles include crosswords and word searches.

A game is played according to a specific set of rules. Game rules should be clear and simple. Using groups of students in teams rather than individual contestants helps involve the entire class.

Guest Speakers

Guest speakers can be recruited from students' families, the school and the community. They provide a valuable link between the classroom and the "real world."

Speakers should be screened before being invited to present to the class. They should have some awareness of the level of student knowledge and should be given direction for the content and focus of the presentation.

Interviewing

Students can interview experts and others about a specific topic either inside or outside of class. Invite experts, family members and others to visit class, or ask students to interview others (family members or friends) outside of class.

Advance preparation for an organized interview session increases the learning potential. A brainstorming session before the interview allows students to develop questions to ask during the interview.

TEACHING STRATEGIES

Oral Presentations

Individual students or groups or panels of students can present information orally to the rest of the class. Such presentations may sometimes involve the use of charts or posters to augment the presentation.

Students enjoy learning and hearing from each other, and the experience stimulates positive interaction. It also helps build students' communication skills.

Encouraging Creative Expression

Student creativity should be encouraged and challenged. Creative expression provides the opportunity to integrate language arts, fine arts and personal experience into a lesson. It also helps meet the diverse needs of students with different learning styles.

Artistic Expression or Creative Writing

Students may be offered a choice of expressing themselves in art or through writing. They may write short stories, poems or letters, or create pictures or collages about topics they are studying. Such a choice accommodates the differing needs and talents of students.

This technique can be used as a follow-up to most lessons. Completed work should be displayed in the classroom, at school or in the community.

Dramatic Presentations

Dramatic presentations may take the form of skits or mock news, radio or television shows. They can be presented to the class or to larger groups in the school or community. When equipment is available, videotapes of these presentations provide an opportunity to present students' work to other classes in the school and other groups in the community.

Such presentations are highly motivating activities, because they actively involve students in learning desired concepts. They also allow students to practice new behaviors in a safe setting and help them personalize information presented in class.

Roleplays

Acting out difficult situations provides students practice in new behaviors in a safe setting. Sometimes students are given a part to play, and other times they are given an idea and asked to improvise. Students need time to decide the central action of the situation and how they will resolve it before they make their presentation. Such activities are highly motivating because they actively involve students in learning desired concepts or practicing certain behaviors.

Sharing Thoughts, Feelings and Opinions

In the sensitive areas of health education, students may have a variety of opinions and feelings. Providing a safe atmosphere in which to discuss opinions and feelings encourages students to share their ideas and listen and learn from others. Such discussion also provides an opportunity to clarify misinformation and correct misconceptions.

Brainstorming

Brainstorming is used to stimulate discussion of an issue or topic. It can be done with the whole class or in smaller groups. It can be used both to gather information and to share thoughts and opinions.

All statements should be accepted without comment or judgment from the teacher or other students. Ideas can be listed on the board, on butcher paper or newsprint or on a transparency. Brainstorming should continue until all ideas have been exhausted or a predetermined time limit has been reached.

Class Discussion

A class discussion led by the teacher or by students is a valuable educational strategy. It can be used to initiate, amplify or summarize a lesson. Such discussions also provide a way to share ideas, opinions and concerns that may have been generated in small group work.

Clustering

Clustering is a simple visual technique that involves diagraming ideas around a main topic. The main topic is written on the board and circled. Other related ideas are then attached to the central idea or to each other with connecting lines.

Clustering can be used as an adjunct to brainstorming. Because there is no predetermined number of secondary ideas, clustering can accommodate all brainstorming ideas.

Continuum Voting

Continuum voting is a stimulating discussion technique. Students express the extent to which they agree or disagree with a statement read by the teacher. The classroom should be prepared for this activity with a sign that says "Agree" on one wall and a sign that says "Disagree" on the opposite wall. There should be room for students to move freely between the 2 signs.

As the teacher reads a statement, students move to a point between the signs that reflects their thoughts or feelings. The closer to the "Agree" sign they stand, the stronger their agreement. The closer to the "Disagree" sign they stand, the stronger their disagreement. A position in the center between the signs indicates a neutral stance.

Dyad Discussion

Working in pairs allows students to provide encouragement and support to each other. Students who may feel uncomfortable sharing in the full class may be more willing to share their thoughts and feelings with 1 other person. Depending on the task, dyads may be temporary, or students may meet regularly with a partner and work together to achieve their goals.

Forced Field Analysis

This strategy is used to discuss an issue that is open to debate. Students analyze a situation likely to be approved by some students and opposed by others. For example, if the subject of discussion was the American diet, some students might support the notion that Americans consume healthy foods because of the wide variety of foods available. Other students might express concern about the amount of foods that are high in sodium, fat and sugar.

Questioning skills are critical to the success of this technique. A good way to open such a discussion is to ask students, "What questions should you ask to determine if you support or oppose this idea?" The pros and cons of students' analysis can be charted on the board or on a transparency.

Journal Writing

Journal writing affords the opportunity for thinking and writing. Expressive writing requires that students become actively involved in the learning process. However, writing may become a less effective tool for learning if students must worry about spelling and punctuation. Students should be encouraged to write freely in their journals, without fear of evaluation.

Panel Discussion

Panel discussions provide an opportunity to discuss different points of view about a health topic, problem or issue. Students can research and develop supporting arguments for different sides. Such research and discussion enhances understanding of content.

Panel members may include experts from the community as well as students. Panel discussions are usually directed by a moderator and may be followed by a question and answer period.

Self-Assessment

Personal inventories provide a tool for self-assessment. Providing privacy around personal assessments allows students to be honest in their responses. Volunteers can share answers or the questions can be discussed in general, but no students should have to share answers they would prefer to keep private. Students can use the information to set personal goals for changing behaviors.

Small Groups

Students working together can help stimulate each other's creativity. Small group activities are cooperative, but have less formal structure than cooperative learning groups. These activities encourage collective thinking and provide opportunities for students to work with others and increase social skills.

Surveys and Inventories

Surveys and inventories can be used to assess knowledge, attitudes, beliefs and practices. These instruments can be used to gather knowledge about a variety of groups, including students, parents and other family members, and teachers.

Students can use surveys others have designed or design their own. When computers are available, students can use them to summarize their information, create graphs and prepare presentations of the data.

Developing Critical Thinking

Critical thinking skills help students analyze health topics and issues. These activities require that students learn to gather information, consider the consequences of actions and behaviors and make responsible decisions. They challenge students to perform higher-level thinking and clearly communicate their ideas.

Case Studies

Case studies provide written histories of a problem or situation. Students can read, discuss and analyze these situations. This strategy encourages student involvement and helps students personalize the health-related concepts presented in class.

TEACHING STRATEGIES

Cooperative Learning Groups

Cooperative learning is an effective teaching strategy that has been shown to have a positive effect on students' achievement and interpersonal skills. Students can work in small groups to disseminate and share information, analyze ideas or solve problems. The size of the group depends on the nature of the lesson and the make-up of the class. Groups work best with from 2–6 members.

Group structure will affect the success of the lessons. Groups can be formed by student choice, random selection, or a more formal, teacher-influenced process. Groups seem to function best when they represent the variety and balance found in the classroom. Groups also work better when each student has a responsibility within the group (reader, recorder, timer, reporter, etc.).

While groups are working on their tasks, the teacher should move from group to group, answering questions and dealing with any problems that arise. At the conclusion of the group process, some closure should take place.

Debates

Students can debate the pros and cons of many issues relating to health. Suggesting that students defend an opposing point of view provides an additional learning experience.

During a debate, each side has the opportunity to present their arguments and to refute each others' arguments. After the debate, class members can choose the side with which they agree.

Factual Writing

Once students have been presented with information about a topic, a variety of writing assignments can challenge them to clarify and express their ideas and opinions. Position papers, letters to the editor, proposals and public service announcements provide a forum in which students can express their opinions, supporting them with facts, figures and reasons.

Media Analysis

Students can analyze materials from a variety of media, including printed matter, music, TV programs, movies, video games and advertisements, to identify health-related messages. Such analysis might include identifying the purpose of the piece, the target audience, underlying messages, motivations and stereotypes.

TEACHING STRATEGIES

Personal Contracts

Personal contracts, individual commitments to changing behavior, can help students make positive changes in their health-related behaviors. The wording of a personal contract may include the behavior to be changed, a plan for changing the behavior and the identification of possible problems and support systems.

However, personal contracts should be used with caution. Behavior change may be difficult, especially in the short term. Students should be encouraged to make personal contracts around goals they are likely to meet.

Research

Research requires students to seek information to complete a task. Students may be given prepared materials that they must use to complete an assignment, or they may have to locate resources and gather information on their own. As part of this strategy, students must compile and organize the information they collect.

GLOSSARY

A

activity—A specific action or motion.

aerobic—The form of energy production in the body that requires the presence of oxygen; used for activities such as walking or jogging.

aerobic activity—Exercise that involves continuous and repetitive movements of the large muscle groups; e.g., jogging, bicycling, skating, cross country skiing, walking and jumping rope.

aerobic capacity—The body's ability to take in and use oxygen so muscles can keep working.

apocrine—A type of sweat gland that contributes to the characteristic odor of perspiration.

B

body composition—The ratio of fat to lean tissue in the body.

body image—The mental picture we have of our physical selves.

C

calisthenics—Exercises done without equipment; e.g., pushups, curl-ups.

carbohydrate—A nutrient composed of carbon, hydrogen and oxygen; the body's preferred form of energy.

cardiorespiratory endurance—The body's ability to take in and use oxygen so that muscles can function; also known as aerobic fitness. It is dependent on cardiorespiratory capacity and the ability of cells in the body to efficiently use oxygen and release carbon dioxide.

complex carbohydrates—A source of vitamins, minerals and energy; found in whole grains, fruits and vegetables.

cool-down—A gradual decrease from vigorous exercise.

F

fat—A nutrient that is a source of energy and that can be stored.

fit—In good physical condition; healthy.

FIT—An acronym for Frequency, Intensity, Time—important concepts in using exercise to improve fitness.

fitness—A combination of qualities that enable an individual to meet the physical demands of life.

flexibility—The elasticity of muscles and connective tissues, which determines the range of motion of the joints.

free weights—Hand-held weights, barbells and dumbbells.

GLOSSARY

frequency—The number of times an action is repeated in a given period.

G

goal—An end that a person aims to reach or accomplish.

H

habit—An act that is done often, in a certain way, and has become automatic.

healthy—Having a state of well-being; defined as physical, intellectual, emotional and social well-being.

hormone—A chemical substance secreted by an endocrine gland and transported in the blood or other body fluids to stimulate growth and regulate activities.

I

insomnia—The inability to sleep.

intensity—A higher-than-normal level of stress that is self-imposed during exercising.

M

mineral—An inorganic substance that plays a vital role in human metabolism.

muscular endurance—The power of muscles to keep on working.

muscular strength—The force that muscles can exert upon contraction for the purpose of bodily movement and support; the ability of muscles to work.

N

nutrient—A chemical substance found in food that the body needs for proper growth and function.

nutrition—The science of food and how it is used in the body.

O

Olympic games—International athletic competition involving a variety of summer and winter sports.

overloading—To demand more work from muscles than is normally required.

P

perspiration—The moisture given off in perspiring; sweat.

physical—Referring to the body.

physical cues—Signals from the body.

plan—An outline; a scheme for making, doing or arranging something; a project; a program; a schedule.

GLOSSARY

protein—A nutrient composed of carbon, hydrogen, oxygen and nitrogen, whose major function is the growth, maintenance and repair of body tissues.

pulse—The regular beating in the arteries, caused by the contractions of the heart.

pulse rate—The number of times the heart beats in a given period.

R

record—The best performance achieved to date.

REM—Rapid eye movement.

REM sleep—The dream stage during sleep, indicated by the back-and-forth movement of the eyes under the eyelids.

rep (repetition)—Each time an exercise movement is completed.

rest—A period of ease and refreshment; relief from anything distressing, disturbing, annoying or tiring; peace of mind.

S

safe—Free from damage, danger or injury.

self-esteem—The way people feel about themselves.

set—Group(s) of repetitions.

skin-fold measurements—A method for measuring body composition that uses calipers to measure the thickness of folds of skin.

sleep—A natural, regularly recurring condition of rest for the body and mind during which there is little or no conscious thought, sensation or movement.

steroids—Drugs that function like the male hormone testosterone.

stretching— Activities designed to loosen connective tissue (tendons and ligaments) and muscles.

supplements—Vitamins, minerals or proteins that are taken in tablet or capsule form.

T

target heart rate—Figure used to determine the number of heartbeats per minute required to improve aerobic capacity.

time—A period during which an action takes place.

V

vigorous—Forceful; powerful; strong; energetic.

vitamin—A chemical substance present in foods that is essential to normal metabolism and helps regulate body functions.

GLOSSARY

W

warm-up—The first portion of a workout, designed to prepare the body for vigorous exercise.

weight machines—Equipment designed to increase muscular strength and endurance.

REFERENCES

American Alliance for Health, Physical Education, Recreation and Dance. 1989. *Physical best.* Reston, VA.

Bouchard, C., et al. 1989. *Exercise, fitness and health: A consensus of current knowledge.* Champaign, IL: Human Kinetics Press.

Cooper, K. H. 1991. *Kid fitness.* New York: Bantam.

Garzino, M. S. 1996. *Comprehensive health for the middle grades: Fitness and hygiene.* Santa Cruz, CA: ETR Associates.

Hamilton, M., et al. 1990. *The Duke University Medical Center book of diet and fitness.* New York: Fawcett Columbine.

Krantzler, N. J., and K. R. Miner. 1994. *Fitness: Health facts.* Santa Cruz, CA: ETR Associates.

Kusinitz, I., and M. Fine. 1987. *Your guide to getting fit.* 2d ed. Mountain View, CA: Mayfield.

Macmillan health encyclopedia: Nutrition and fitness. 1989. New York: Macmillan.

McArdle, W. D., F. I. Katch and V. L. Katch. 1991. *Exercise physiology: Energy, nutrition and human performance.* Philadelphia: Lea and Febiger.

Mishra, R. 1991. Steroids and sports are a losing proposition. *FDA Consumer* 25 (7): 25-27.

Papenfuss, R. 1994. Physical fitness: A vital component for total health and high-level wellness. In *The comprehensive school health challenge: Promoting health through education,* vol. 1, ed. P. Cortese and K. Middleton, 491-521. Santa Cruz, CA: ETR Associates.

Sharkey, B. J. 1990. *Physiology of fitness.* 3d ed. Champaign, IL: Human Kinetics Books.

Stang, L., and K. R. Miner. 1994. *Nutrition: Health facts.* Santa Cruz, CA: ETR Associates.

Williams, M. H. 1990. *Lifetime fitness and wellness.* Dubuque, IA: Wm. C. Brown.

CONTENTS

Fitness Is...

Name _____ Date _____ Period _____

 DIRECTIONS Look at the word *Fitness* in the center of the page. Brainstorm some words that come to mind when you think of fitness. Write these words around the word *Fitness*. Circle each word you write and draw lines to connect the words. Write down all the words you think of—don't stop to judge your ideas.

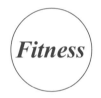

Fitness

FITNESS IS... EXAMPLE

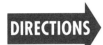 **DIRECTIONS** Look at the word *Fitness* in the center of the page. Brainstorm some words that come to mind when you think of fitness. Write these words around the word *Fitness*. Circle each word you write and draw lines to connect the words. Write down all the words you think of—don't stop to judge your ideas.

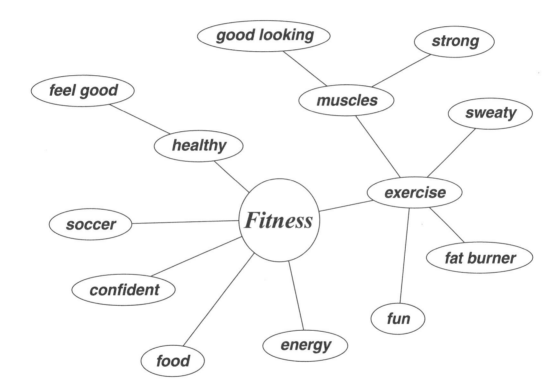

BENEFITS OF FITNESS

Name _____ Date _____ Period _____

DIRECTIONS ▶ Fill in the 3 benefits of fitness that are most important to you. Rank them in order of importance—1 is most important, 3 is least. Then answer the questions.

Benefits of fitness:

1.

2.

3.

Why did you choose these benefits?

How would these benefits improve your life?

FITNESS FACTS

Name _____ Date _____ Period _____

DIRECTIONS ▶ Write a definition of each of these elements of fitness.

Aerobic Capacity

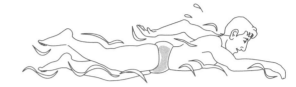

Body Composition

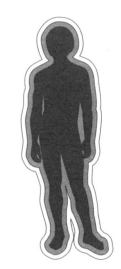

Flexibility

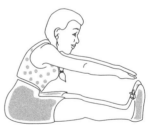

Muscular Strength and Endurance

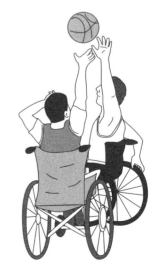

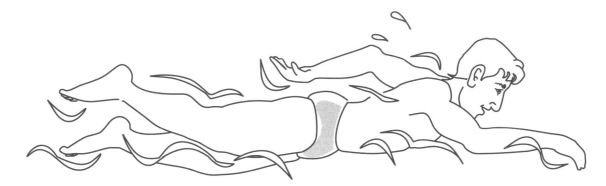

Aerobic Capacity

The body's ability to take in and use oxygen so muscles can keep working.

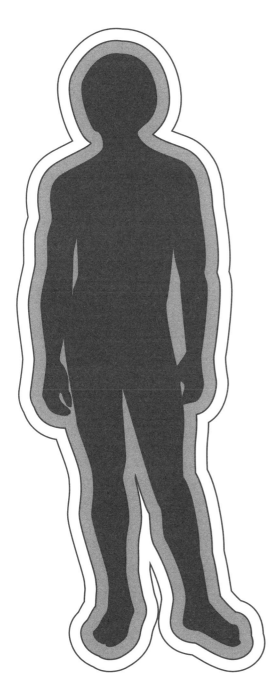

Body Composition

The ratio of fat to lean tissue in the body.

(continued...)

CONTINUED

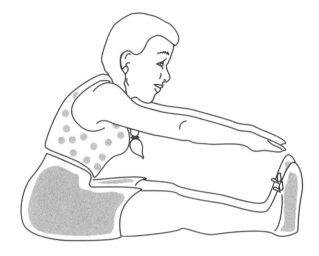

Flexibility

The ability of joints and muscles to move through their full range of motion.

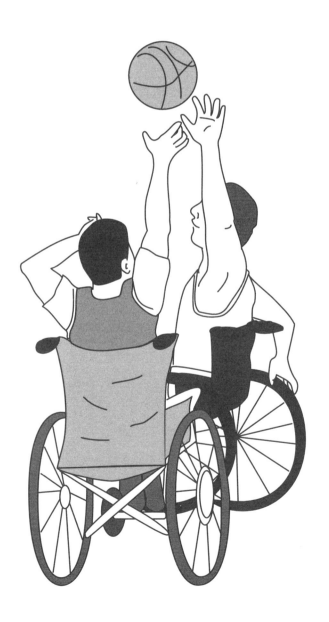

Muscular Strength and Endurance

The ability of muscles to work and to keep on working.

FITNESS CHOICE INVENTORY

Name _____ Date _____ Period _____

DIRECTIONS Answer yes or no to the following questions. Then add your points to determine your level of physical activity.

_____ 1. I usually walk to and from school (at least 1/2 mile each way). (1 point)

_____ 2. I take the stairs instead of elevators or escalators. (1 point)

_____ 3. My daily routine involves:

            _____ a. sitting at school or watching TV at home (0 points)

            _____ b. some physical activity during or after school (4 points)

            _____ c. several hours of heavy sports or work activity (7 points)

_____ 4. I ride my bike or walk to after-school activities (1 point)

_____ 5. I do yard work or housework several hours each week (2 points)

_____ 6. I go to a dance at least once a week. (2 points)

_____ 7. I exercise when I'm feeling stressed. (2 points)

_____ 8. I do stretching exercises several times each week. (3 points)

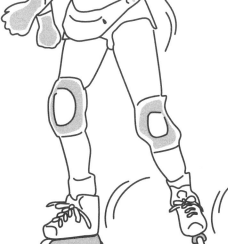

(continued…)

CONTINUED

_____ 9. I perform sit-ups, pull-ups or other exercises 2 or more times a week, for at least 10 minutes per session. **(3 points)**

_____ 10. I lift weights or use exercise equipment:

       _____ a. about once a week **(2 points)**

       _____ b. about twice a week **(4 points)**

       _____ c. 3 times a week **(7 points)**

_____ 11. I engage in a vigorous fitness activity like jogging, aerobic dance or basketball (at least 20 continuous minutes per session):

       _____ a. about once a week **(3 points)**

       _____ b. about twice a week **(5 points)**

       _____ c. at least 3 times per week **(9 points)**

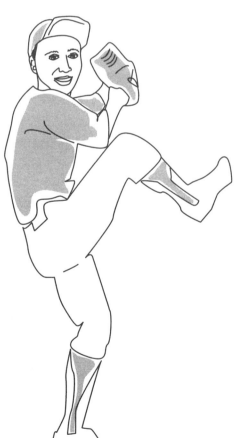

SCORING:

Give yourself the number of points indicated for each *Yes* answer. Then total your points to determine your score.

0 to 7 points— Inactive. Becoming more active will help reduce your risk of health problems.

8 to 14 points— Moderately active. This amount of activity will not maintain your present level of fitness.

15 to 25 points— Active. This amount of activity will maintain an acceptable level of fitness.

26 points or over— Very active. This amount of activity will maintain a high level of fitness.

FITNESS INTERVIEW

Name _____ Date _____ Period _____

DIRECTIONS Interview someone who has exercised regularly for at least 1 year. Write their answers to these questions on this page.

1. What exercise(s) do you do on a regular basis?

2. How long have you been exercising regularly?

3. What is your weekly exercise schedule?

4. Why do you exercise regularly?

5. Do you drink water before, during or after you exercise?

6. What special equipment or clothing (if any) do you use?

7. What are your eating habits? Do you avoid any foods or eat any special foods?

8. How much sleep do you usually get?

9. What advice would you give to someone who wanted to begin a regular exercise program?

MY BODY IMAGE

Name _____ Date _____ Period _____

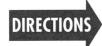 **DIRECTIONS** Rate the parts of your body by placing a number in the blank beside each body part. Use the following scale:

1 – I really like this.
2 – I am satisfied with this.
3 – I have no feelings about this.

4 – I don't like this but can live with it.
5 – I don't like this and would like to change it.

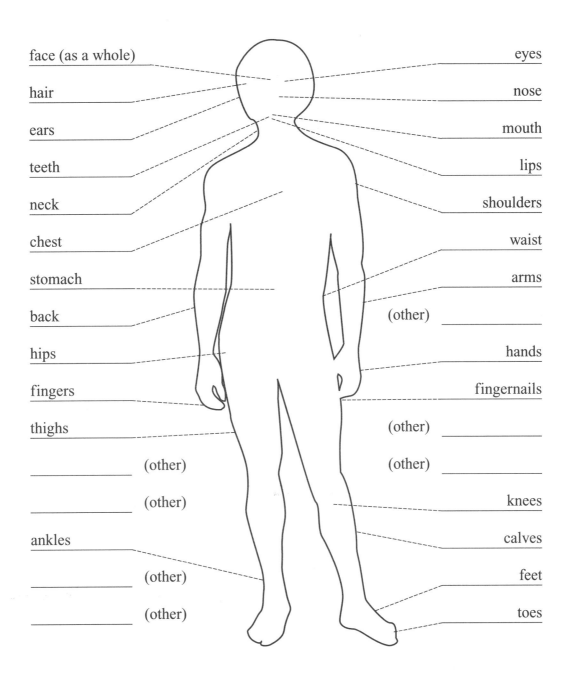

face (as a whole) _____

hair _____

ears _____

teeth _____

neck _____

chest _____

stomach _____

back _____

hips _____

fingers _____

thighs _____

_____ (other)

_____ (other)

ankles _____

_____ (other)

_____ (other)

eyes _____

nose _____

mouth _____

lips _____

shoulders _____

waist _____

arms _____

(other) _____

hands _____

fingernails _____

(other) _____

(other) _____

knees _____

calves _____

feet _____

toes _____

Choosing Health High School

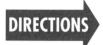
CASE STUDIES

Name _____ Date _____ Period _____

DIRECTIONS ➤ Read and discuss the case studies with your group.

JENNY

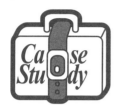

I'm barely 5 feet tall and always thought I would grow at least a few more inches. But now that I'm 18 years old, I realize I'm going to be short like my grandmother on my mother's side of the family. So now I have a choice. I can think of myself as short and shrimpy, or I can think of myself as petite. I think I'll consider myself petite!

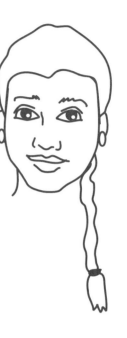

Analysis of Jenny

Jenny wishes she were taller but realizes this is not possible. What are her choices? She can:

• Refuse to accept her height and feel bad about her appearance.

• Accept her height and work on feeling good about herself.

(continued...)

WHAT CAN'T BE CHANGED

CONTINUED

CLINT

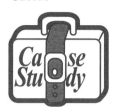

Ever since I was a little kid, I've noticed my mouth is kind of crooked. When I smile, it looks like I'm only smiling with one side of my mouth. This used to really bother me, and I would stand in front of the mirror and practice trying to straighten out my smile.

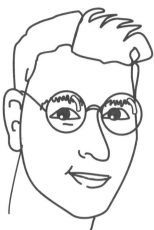

When I was in the ninth grade, I met Michelle. One night at the movies, I made a comment about my crooked mouth. Do you know what she said? She told me that one thing she really liked about me was my crooked smile! She said it made me different from everyone else.

Analysis of Clint

Sometimes we dislike the physical features that we consider different. Clint was surprised to learn that the feature he disliked was actually a feature that made him more attractive to someone he cared about.

Do you think Michelle's reaction to Clint will help change his opinion about his crooked mouth? Do you feel other people notice our faults more or less than we do?

WILLING TO CHANGE

CASE STUDIES

Name _____ Date _____ Period _____

DIRECTIONS ➤ Read and discuss the case studies with your group.

SERGIO

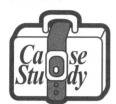

For the past couple of years, I've been self-conscious about my shoulders and chest. They seem underdeveloped compared to the rest of my body. I am most self-conscious when I take my shirt off around other people, like in P. E. class or at the swimming pool.

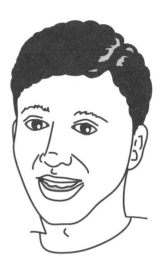

Sometimes I imagine what my body would look like if I had some muscles in my chest and shoulders to kind of balance me out. I believe I would feel better about myself if I did something about the way I look.

Analysis of Sergio

Sergio is dissatisfied with the upper part of his body. What are Sergio's choices? He can:

• Do nothing and continue to be dissatisfied with his appearance.

• Keep the same behavior and change the way he thinks and feels about his chest and shoulders.

• Change his behavior.

What advice would you give Sergio? What behavior must he be willing to change?

(continued...)

WILLING TO CHANGE

CONTINUED

BRANDI

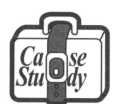

Every time I wear shorts or go shopping for new clothes, I feel fat. If I could just firm up, I could wear the kind of clothes I want to wear. I've thought about beginning an exercise program, so I can look fantastic for the junior prom.

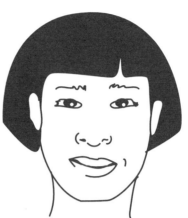

I saw this great black and white dress that would be just perfect. It would look great on me if I could tone up my muscles. I have 6 months until the prom.

Analysis of Brandi

Brandi believes she would look better in the kinds of clothes she wants to wear if she could tone up her muscles. What are her choices? She can:

*   Do nothing and continue to feel bad about her appearance.

*   Keep the same behavior and change the way she thinks and feels about her body. For example, she could buy a different dress that she likes just as well.

*   Change her behavior.

What advice would you give Brandi? What behavior must she be willing to change?

BODY IMAGE ASSESSMENT

Name _____ Date _____ Period _____

DIRECTIONS → Refer to your ratings on the **My Body Image** activity sheet to complete the following paragraph. Fill in the blanks and circle the responses that are most true for you.

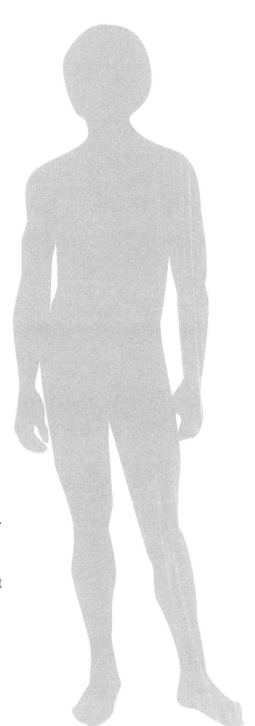

When I look in a full-length mirror, I usually notice my _____ first. This is because I (like, dislike) this part of my body. My best physical feature is my _____. This feature is most attractive because of its (size, shape, color, texture, smell). The part of my body that needs improvement is my _____. If this part of my body were changed, I (would, would not) feel better about myself.

When someone sees me for the first time, the first thing they will notice about my physical appearance is my _____. I am (glad, unhappy) they notice this feature. When I communicate with others, I use my (hands, eyes, body, face) to express my feelings. When I am under stress, my (head, stomach, skin, heart, lungs, _____) is/are the first part of my body to be affected.

Overall, I am (happy, satisfied, unconcerned, somewhat dissatisfied, unhappy) with my body. When thinking about my body, I am most likely to (admire it, worry about it, criticize it, care for it). I am least likely to (enjoy it, look at it, display it, forget about it).

PARTNER PORTRAIT

Name _____ Date _____ Period _____

DIRECTIONS ➤ Read the following paragraph. Then create a portrait of one of your partner's most attractive physical features. The portrait can be a written description or a picture you draw. When you've finished your portrait, answer the questions.

EXAMPLE: MARLA'S EYES

Marla's best feature is her eyes. They are big and brown and surrounded by dark eyelashes. When she smiles, her eyes seem to get bigger and shinier. Marla's eyes are the first thing I noticed about her. I like the way they crinkle up at the corners when she smiles. Marla's eyes are attractive because they are so dark. They seem to help her express what she is saying or feeling.

YOUR PARTNER

THE PORTRAIT

QUESTIONS

1. Why did you choose this feature?

2. Why is this feature attractive?

CHANGING MY BODY IMAGE

Name _____ Date _____ Period _____

PART 1

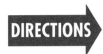 In and around the body outline, describe both positive and negative feelings you have about your body image.

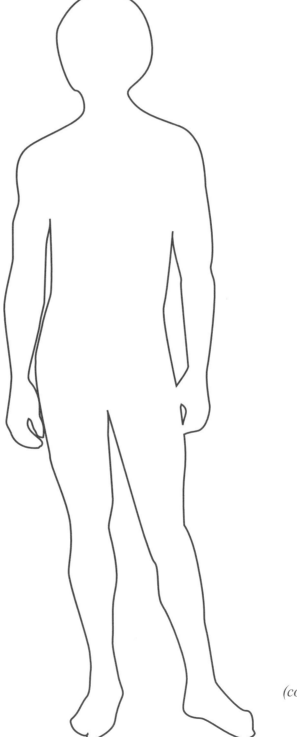

(continued...)

CHANGING MY BODY IMAGE

CONTINUED

PART 2

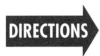 Complete the following statements.

1. I have decided to enhance my body image by

2. My ultimate goal is

3. These are the steps I can take to reach my goal:
    a.

    b.

4. Describe your feelings when your partner described one of your most attractive features.

5. Write what you said after your partner finished reading his or her description. How did you accept the compliment?

6. Identify 3 feelings you have about your body.

ROLEPLAY CARDS

PAT

 Roleplay this situation:

You have a new haircut that looks great on you. When Tracy notices and compliments you, you smile and say, "Thanks, I'm glad you like it."

TRACY

 Roleplay this situation:

You are in health class and notice Pat's new haircut. You walk over to Pat and say, "Pat, your hair is way cool. It really makes you look good."

ASSESS YOUR FITNESS

Name _____ Date _____ Period _____

DIRECTIONS ➤ Fill in your scores on each of the assessments.

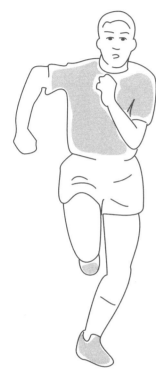

AEROBIC CAPACITY
One Mile Walk/Run
time=_____:_____ (minutes:seconds)

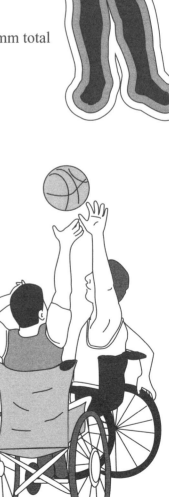

BODY COMPOSITION
Sum of Skinfolds
triceps _____mm + calf _____mm = _____mm total

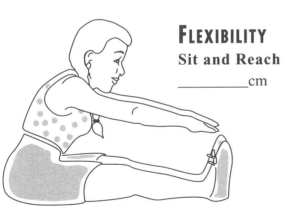

FLEXIBILITY
Sit and Reach
_____cm

MUSCULAR STRENGTH AND ENDURANCE
Sit-Ups
number performed _____

Pull-Ups
number performed _____

Choosing Health High School

How Fit Are You?

GIRLS

Age	Activity				
	Walk/Run (min.)	Skinfolds (mm)	Sit & Reach (cm)	Sit-ups	Pull-ups
12	11:00	16–36	25	33	1
13	10:30	16–36	25	33	1
14	10:30	16–36	25	35	1
15	10:30	16–36	25	35	1
16	10:30	16–36	25	35	1
17	10:30	16–36	25	35	1
18	10:30	16–36	25	35	1
	aerobic capacity	body composition	flexibility	muscular strength and endurance	

BOYS

Age	Activity				
	Walk/Run (min.)	Skinfolds (mm)	Sit & Reach (cm)	Sit-ups	Pull-ups
12	9:00	12–25	25	38	2
13	8:00	12–25	25	40	3
14	7:45	12–25	25	40	4
15	7:30	12–25	25	42	5
16	7:30	12–25	25	44	5
17	7:30	12–25	25	44	5
18	7:30	12–25	25	44	5
	aerobic capacity	body composition	flexibility	muscular strength and endurance	

Frequency—3 to 6 Times Each Week
Intensity—At Your Target Heart Rate
Time—At Least 20 Minutes
Type of Activity—Continuous and Repetitive

Some Popular Aerobic Activities

aerobic dance	skateboarding	swimming
ballet	skating	tennis
basketball	skiing	volleyball
bicycling	soccer	walking
gymnastics		
jogging		
jumping rope		
karate		
racquetball		
rowing		

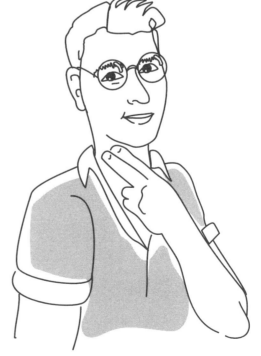

Checking Your Pulse

Your Target Heart Rate

Name _____ Date _____ Period _____

220

− _____ your age

= _____ maximum heart rate

− _____ your r.h.r.
(resting heart rate)

= _____

× .70

= _____

+ _____ your r.h.r.

= _____ upper end of your
target heart rate

220

− _____ your age

= _____ maximum heart rate

− _____ your r.h.r.
(resting heart rate)

= _____

× .50

= _____

+ _____ your r.h.r.

= _____ lower end of your
target heart rate

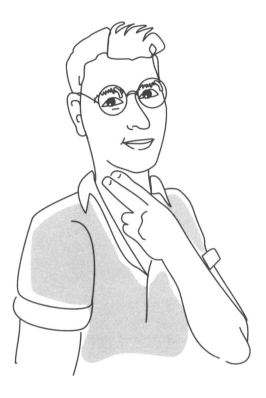

Choosing Health High School

PERSONAL PLAN EXAMPLE

I _____ ***Betty Hubbard*** _____ can
(first name, last name)

_____ ***maintain*** _____ my aerobic capacity by:
(improve, maintain)

1. Warm up: _____ ***walking*** _____ for ____ *5* ____ minutes
(enter your warm-up activity)   (#)

2. S T R E T C H I N G for ____ *5* ____ minutes
(#)

3. Aerobic activity: _____ ***jogging*** _____

   at my target heart rate of ___ ***156–168*** ___ beats/minute for ____ *25* ____ minutes
   (enter your THR)   (#)

4. Cool down: _____ ***walking*** _____ for ____ *5* ____ minutes
(enter your cool down activity)   (#)

5. S T R E T C H I N G for ____ *5* ____ minutes
(#)

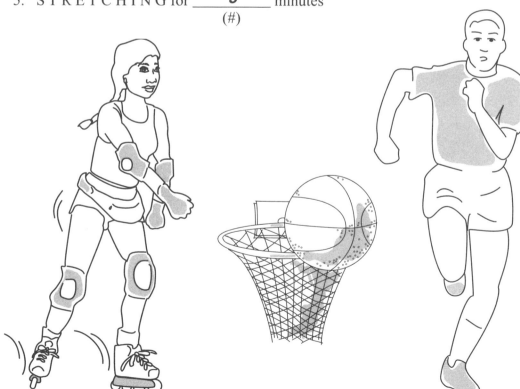

Choosing Health High School

Personal Plan

Name _____ Date _____ Period _____

I _____ can
  (first name, last name)

_____ my aerobic capacity by:
  (improve, maintain)

1. Warm up: _____ for _____ minutes
             (enter your warm-up activity)   (#)

2. S T R E T C H I N G for _____ minutes
                          (#)

3. Aerobic activity: _____

   at my target heart rate of _____ beats/minute for _____ minutes
                (enter your THR)   (#)

4. Cool down: _____ for _____ minutes
              (enter your cool down activity)   (#)

5. S T R E T C H I N G for _____ minutes
                          (#)

Choosing Health High School

Exercises for Flexibility

Neck Stretch

Shoulder Rolls

Straddle Stretch

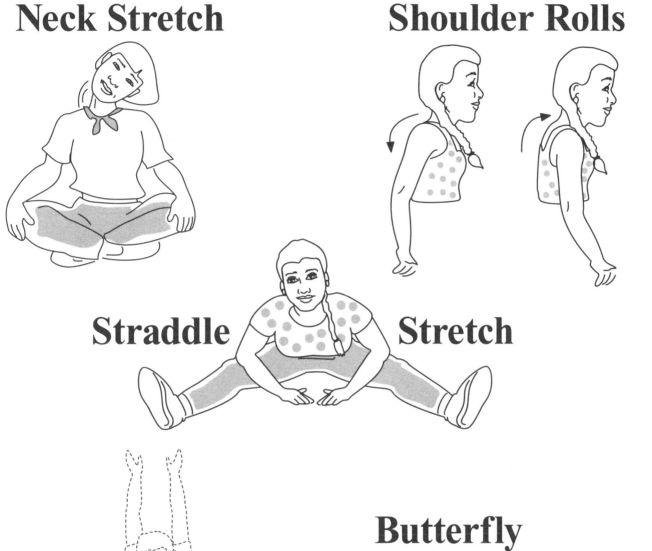

Body Circle

Butterfly Stretch

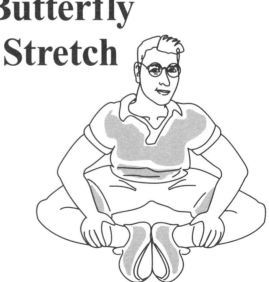

IMPROVING FLEXIBILITY

Name _____ Date _____ Period _____

Neck stretch (for neck)—Take head from right or left side, forward, and around to the other side. Reverse. Turn head from side to side. Do not tip head backward.

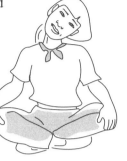

Shoulder rolls (for shoulders)—Make smooth circles with shoulders. Keep arms down at sides. Circle in both directions.

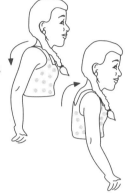

Body circle (for hips, spine, legs)—Bend knees then reach arms in a continuous circle overhead, to the side, floor and back up. Keep the head up.

Butterfly stretch (for inner thighs)—Bring heels together and toward the body. Grab ankles and press knees toward the floor. Stretch the torso forward.

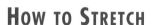

Straddle stretch (for legs and lower back)—Stretch forward with upper body between open legs. Keep knees facing up and legs and back straight.

HOW TO STRETCH

When stretching:
*   Reach to the point of discomfort, then back off slightly.
*   Relax and hold the stretch for 10–20 seconds.
*   Concentrate on the feeling of the stretch. The stretch should never be painful.

GUIDELINES FOR SAFE STRETCHING

*   Before stretching, increase your body temperature by running in place slowly or doing some other rhythmic activity. Raising body temperature increases flexibility and reduces the risk of injury.
*   Do a minimum of 5 repetitions of each stretch.
*   Breathe slowly and rhythmically throughout the stretches.
*   Perform each stretch regularly. If you don't use it, you lose it.
*   Don't do any unsafe exercises. For example, twisting hops, gymnastic bridges, straight-leg toe touches, deep knee bends, and straight leg sit-ups can injure the knees and back.

High Jumper

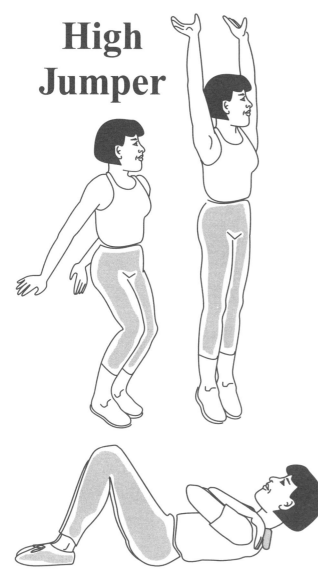

Inner-Thigh Raise

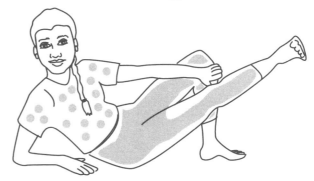

Sit-Ups

Push-Ups (modified)

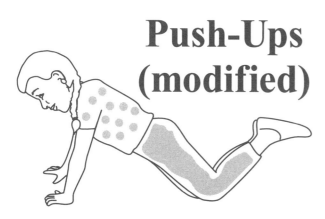

Push-Ups (advanced)

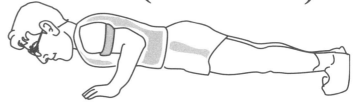

IMPROVING STRENGTH AND ENDURANCE

Name _____ Date _____ Period _____

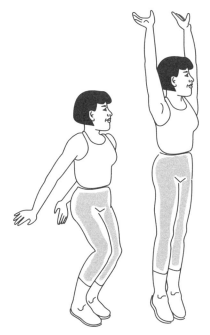

High jumper (for hips and upper and lower legs)—Start with knees slightly bent. Jump as high as possible while raising both arms.

Outer-thigh raise (for outer thigh and hip)—Rest on forearm and hip, with bottom leg bent at a 90-degree angle and top leg raised slightly. Slowly lift and lower top leg in a straight line with body. Repeat with the other leg.

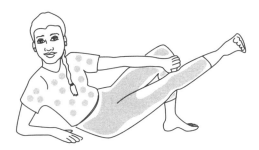

Sit-ups (for abdominals)—Lie on back with knees flexed and feet on the floor. Place heels 12 to 18 inches from the buttocks. Cross arms on the chest with hands on opposite shoulders. Tuck chin toward the chest. Tighten abdominal muscles to curl shoulders and upper back off the floor. Keep feet on the floor.

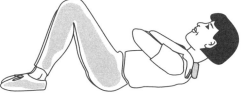

Inner-thigh raise (for inner thighs)—Rest on hip with forearm and bent upper leg helping you balance. Rotate bottom leg out so that heel is turned up and toes are turned down. Keep foot flexed and lift leg as high as you can without rolling your hip back. Repeat with the other leg.

Push-ups (modified) (for chest, shoulders and arms)—Assume a front-leaning position with knees bent up and hands under shoulders. Lower the chest toward the floor. Raise and repeat.

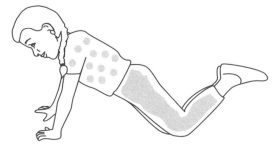

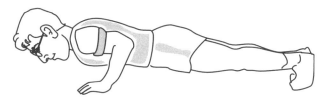

Push-ups (advanced) (for chest, shoulders and arms)—Assume a front-leaning position. Lower the chest toward the floor. Raise and repeat.

(continued...)

Choosing Health High School

CONTINUED

REPS AND SETS

Reps and sets are the building blocks of the workout. Reps are repetitions of an exercise. To do a sit-up for 8 reps means to perform it 8 times in a row before resting. A set is 1 group of reps followed by a rest interval. Performing 8 sit-ups, resting 45 seconds to a minute, then doing 8 more sit-ups equals 2 sets.

A workout for muscular strength or endurance should include 5–12 reps of each exercise for 3 sets. When an exercise becomes easy to do, add 2-1/2 to 5 pounds to the barbell, dumbbells or other equipment.

GUIDELINES FOR SAFELY IMPROVING MUSCULAR STRENGTH AND ENDURANCE

- Have an exercise instructor demonstrate the proper use of the equipment if you are using free weights or machines.
- Don't exercise alone. Use a spotter if you're using barbells.
- Warm up and stretch before beginning.
- Gradually increase your level of exercise.
- Allow at least 48 hours for your muscles to recover from a workout. Workouts on consecutive days do more harm than good, because the body cannot adapt that quickly.
- Don't let more than 4 days pass without working out. Muscles will begin to break down if you let more than 3 or 4 days pass without exercising them.
- Inhale when lifting and exhale when releasing.

FITNESS FOCUS

Name _____ Date _____ Period _____

DIRECTIONS → Read the following case studies. Discuss the case studies with your group and decide which element of fitness each person needs to improve. Then write an exercise prescription for each person. List specific ways in which the element of fitness can be improved.

CLEO

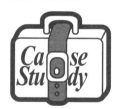

Cleo had been excited about the big Christmas dance for weeks, because Julio had asked her to go with him. The band was great and all her friends were there. The decorations looked terrific, and Julio and Cleo were having a great time.

But after about 30 minutes of nonstop dancing, Cleo had to sit out some of the dances. She couldn't catch her breath. She just didn't seem to have the energy to keep going.

Element of fitness that needs improvement:

Fitness prescription:

RAPHAEL

School was almost over, and Raphael was looking forward to some lazy afternoons with friends at the lake. He got his swimsuit from his bottom drawer and pulled it on. Uh oh! The suit seemed to be a little tighter this year. Raphael decided to take a look in the mirror. Oops! He noticed a few bulges and ripples that weren't there last year.

Raphael was concerned about his appearance. In only a couple of months, the lake would be warm enough for swimming.

Element of fitness that needs improvement:

Fitness prescription:

(continued...)

FITNESS FOCUS

CONTINUED

NIKKI

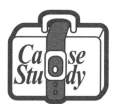

Nikki is pregnant with her first baby. She's very excited. But lately, Nikki has developed a backache that just won't go away. She bent over the other day to pick up a book and had trouble straightening up.

Element of fitness that needs improvement:

Fitness prescription:

LEONA

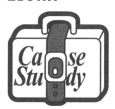

Leona has always helped her neighbors out and earned a little spending money by raking leaves in the fall. This October, Leona discovered that she got tired before she finished raking the first yard. The next day she was so sore she could hardly get out of bed.

Element of fitness that needs improvement:

Fitness prescription:

MITCH

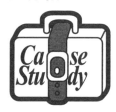

Mitch had been bragging about the used car he bought from his cousin. It had a great sound system and a new paint job. Mitch drove his new car to the Yogurt Factory for a waffle cone. When he was ready to leave, he couldn't get the car started. He tried to push the car while his girlfriend steered, but it wouldn't budge.

Element of fitness that needs improvement:

Fitness prescription:

FACILITY OR PROGRAM SURVEY

Name _____ Date _____ Period _____

DIRECTIONS ▶ Visit or call a fitness facility or program in your community. Then answer the following questions.

1. What is the name of the facility or program you visited or called?

2. Is it public or private?

3. Where is it located?

4. What hours is the facility open? (For programs, what is the time available for the program?)

5. What are the costs involved?

6. Are supervisors or instructors present? What kind of training do they have?

7. Are there facilities or classes available for aerobic workouts? (Circle all that are available.)

    treadmills   jogging/walking track

    Stairmasters   aerobic dance floor

    stationary bicycles   aerobics classes (list them)

    swimming pool   other

    Nordic track

(continued…)

CONTINUED

8. Does the facility or program offer regular monitoring of these things? (Circle all that are available.)

blood pressure   aerobic capacity

cholesterol levels   triglycerides

body composition   muscular strength and endurance

flexibility   other

9. Are users encouraged to attend at least 3 or more times each week?

10. What different kinds of classes are offered? (aerobic dance, nutrition, stress management, swimming, etc.)

11. Are there adequate dressing rooms, showers and lockers available? (Circle all that apply.)

showers

dressing rooms

lockers

12. Based on your visit, describe the positives and negatives of this facility or program.

AN OVERHEARD CONVERSATION

Name _____ Date _____ Period _____

 DIRECTIONS Some common beliefs about fitness are highlighted in the following conversation. With your group, decide whether each statement is true or false. Circle the statements you think are true.

Mark: Hey, are you guys running in the 10K this weekend?

Susan: I'm thinking about it. But I've never run in a race before, so I'm kind of nervous.

Lauren: I've signed up. I heard ***it's going to be hot, but I've got this great looking black bodysuit to wear!*** That's why I'm taking a couple of salt tablets just in case. You know, ***when you sweat, your body needs the extra salt.***

Susan: Is that true? I always thought that ***if you sweat a lot, you need to drink some of those drinks that you see advertised on TV.*** You know, the ones with the special chemicals in them.

Matt: I'm already in training for the race. I've been ***taking extra vitamins and a high protein powder to make sure my body has the protein it needs to make lots of muscle.*** Everybody knows that's important if you're trying to get in shape. And about 10 minutes before the race, I'll ***eat 2 candy bars to give me the quick energy I need for that extra edge.***

Mark: My dad says ***carbohydrates are the foods to eat when you exercise.*** He should know. One of the guys he works with is a bodybuilder. You should see this guy! He's so big that he has to get his clothes at a special store.

(continued…)

CONTINUED

Lauren: I'll bet your dad's friend takes steroids. I've heard *steroids are really dangerous.* I read in the newspaper about a man who grew breasts after he took steroids and a teenager who got a liver disease!

Matt: I don't believe that garbage. *Steroids only make your muscles grow faster and stronger.* No one would take them if they did weird things to your body.

Susan: Who knows about that stuff? I'd like to go with you guys, but I don't have any running shoes.

Mark: Just wear those shoes you have on. *Your shoes really don't matter.* You're not running the Boston Marathon.

Susan: I've got to go. See you guys this weekend. Be sure to get rested up for the 10K. You know, *you need 2–3 extra hours of sleep when you're a high-powered athlete.*

PLANNING FOR FITNESS

#1. The right clothes make exercise more enjoyable and reduce the risk of weather-related problems.

#2. Drinking water is the best way to replace the fluids lost during physical activity.

#3. A balanced diet provides adequate nutrition for the demands of physical activity.

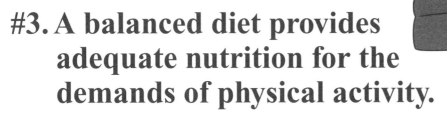

#4. Steroid use can damage body organs and cause psychological changes.

#5. Proper exercise equipment decreases wear and tear on the body and reduces the risk of injury.

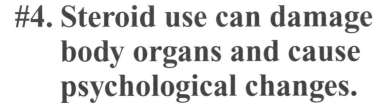

#6. Adequate sleep prepares the body for physical activity and contributes to overall fitness.

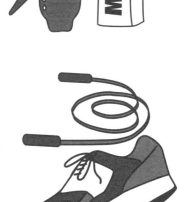

Choosing Health High School

Brain

Increased hostility can lead to tranquilizer use, hypertension, psychological dependence and eating compulsions; increases aggression, which makes injuries more probable.

Face

Facial hair growth, body hair growth and baldness in women; acne in both men and women.

Heart

High blood pressure, clogging of arteries.

Genitals

Sterility or atrophied testicles in men; menstrual irregularities, enlarged genitals in women.

Throat

Deepening of voice in women.

Chest

Breast growth in men; breast cancer and decreased breast size in women.

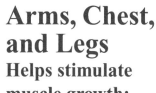

Arms, Chest, and Legs

Helps stimulate muscle growth; decreases recovery time needed between workouts.

Liver and Prostate

Liver cancer in men and women; prostate cancer in men.

RUNNING THE 10K

Name _____ Date _____ Period _____

 DIRECTIONS With your group, answer the following questions about preparing to run the 10K.

It's a cold winter Saturday morning. You are up early getting ready for the 10K. The weather channel forecasts clear skies with a high of 38 degrees. The 10K will start at 10:00 a.m.

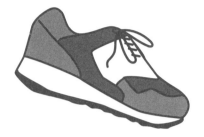

1. How should you dress?

2. What should you eat before the run?

3. What should you drink before, during and after the run?

4. Is there any equipment you should take with you?

5. What advice would you give to a friend who wants to start a regular exercise program?

    a. about nutrition?

    b. about sleep?

    c. about taking steroids?

Name _____ Date _____ Period _____

DIRECTIONS With your group, answer the following questions about preparing to hike
Pinnacle Mountain.

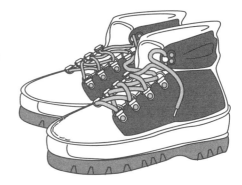

It's a cool spring morning. You are preparing to hike
Pinnacle Mountain with a group of friends. The hike
takes about 3 hours to complete. The weather
channel forecasts overcast skies with a chance of
rain. The expected high for the day is 50 degrees.
You are to meet your friends at 1:00 p.m.

1. How should you dress?

2. What should you eat before the hike?

3. What should you drink before, during and after the hike?

4. Is there any equipment you should take with you?

5. What advice would you give to a friend who wants to start a regular exercise
   program?

   a. about nutrition?

   b. about sleep?

   c. about taking steroids?

PLAYING IN THE HOOPFEST

Name _____ Date _____ Period _____

DIRECTIONS ▶ With your group, answer the following questions about preparing to play in the Hoopfest.

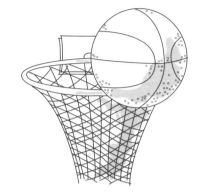

It's a hot summer day. You are preparing to play in the city's Hoopfest (3-on-3 basketball) with a group of friends. The weather channel forecasts sunny skies with high humidity. The expected high for the day is 90 degrees. The first game starts at 9:00 a.m., with additional games scheduled throughout the day.

1. How should you dress?

2. What should you eat before the game?

3. What should you drink before, during and after the game?

4. Is there any equipment you should take with you?

5. What advice would you give you a friend who wants to start a regular exercise program?

    a. about nutrition?

    b. about sleep?

    c. about taking steroids?

SETTING FITNESS GOALS

Name _____ Date _____ Period _____

 DIRECTIONS Consider the following list of fitness goals. Check yes if the goal is a reason you would give for beginning a fitness program. Check no if the goal is not your personal reason for fitness.

I would like to:

	Yes	No
1. Reduce my risk of disease.	☐	☐
2. Have a stronger heart.	☐	☐
3. Have a more positive outlook.	☐	☐
4. Reduce or control the amount of stress I feel.	☐	☐
5. Feel better about myself.	☐	☐
6. Improve my digestion.	☐	☐
7. Increase my energy level.	☐	☐
8. Lower my body fat.	☐	☐
9. Improve my appearance.	☐	☐
10. Sleep better and feel more rested.	☐	☐
11. Lower my blood pressure.	☐	☐
12. Live longer.	☐	☐
13. Have a healthier immune system.	☐	☐
14. Lower my cholesterol level.	☐	☐
15. Reduce my risk of injury.	☐	☐

RATINGS FOR POPULAR ACTIVITIES

ACTIVITIES

ELEMENTS	Jogging	Bicycling	Swimming	Skating (in-line)	Racquet sports	Cross-country skiing	Rope skipping	Step aerobics	Hiking	Aerobics (moderate impact)	Walking
Aerobic capacity	3–5	2–5	3–5	2–4	2–4	4–5	3–5	2–4	2–4	2–4	1–2
Muscular strength and endurance	1–3	2–3	3	3	3	4	3	3	1–3	2–3	1–2
Flexibility	1	1	2	2	3	2	1–2	3	1	2–3	1
Body composition	5	3	3	3	3	4–5	3–5	3–4	3	3	3

1 = low   2 = fair   3 = average   4 = good   5 = excellent

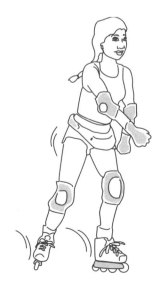
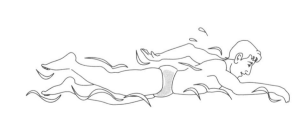
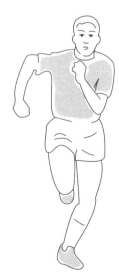

DEVELOPING YOUR FITNESS PLAN

Name _____ Date _____ Period _____

DIRECTIONS ▸ Use these steps to set a personal fitness goal for yourself. Developing a plan will help you reach your goal.

1. Make it personal. Write down the element(s) of fitness you most want to improve.

2. Motivate yourself. Write down the most important goal you expect to achieve.

3. Choose activities you will continue. Write down the activities you choose.

4. Proceed gradually. Write a reasonable and attainable exercise plan.

5. Plan for fitness. List the times you have available for exercise and the equipment you will need.

6. Choose your reward. Make a list of healthy activities you enjoy.

DEVELOPING YOUR FITNESS PLAN EXAMPLE

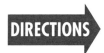 **DIRECTIONS** Use these steps to set a personal fitness goal for yourself. Developing a plan will help you reach your goal.

1. Make it personal. Write down the element(s) of fitness you most want to improve.
   body composition and aerobic capacity

2. Motivate yourself. Write down the most important goal you expect to achieve.
   to improve my appearance

3. Choose activities you will continue. Write down the activities you choose.
   walking, jogging and aerobic dance

4. Proceed gradually. Write a reasonable and attainable exercise plan.
   Warm up by walking around the block.
   Stretch by doing flexibility exercises.
   Jog for 20 minutes at my THR.
   Cool down by walking.
   Stretch again.

5. Plan for fitness. List the times you have available for exercise and the equipment you will need.
   after school on Tuesday and Thursday
   Saturday or Sunday afternoon
   shorts and a T-shirt
   jogging shoes

6. Choose your reward. Make a list of healthy activities you enjoy.
   going to the movies with friends
   talking on the phone
   driving the car

Fitness Plan

Name _____   Date _____   Period _____

Week of: _____

Goal for the week:

Day	Activity	Time	Equipment	Reward
Sunday				
Monday				
Tuesday				
Wednesday				
Thursday				
Friday				
Saturday				

Choosing Health High School

FITNESS PLAN EXAMPLE

Week of: _____ *April 22–28* _____

Goal for the week:
Increase amount of jogging time to 25 minutes.
Spend 5 minutes stretching after jogging.

Day	Activity	Time	Equipment	Reward
Sunday	Walk to Carrie's	afternoon	comfortable shoes	talk to Carrie
Monday	Stretch—warm-up—jog 25 minutes—cool down—stretch	afternoon	jogging shoes, shorts and shirt	hot shower
Tuesday	none	none	none	——
Wednesday	Stretch—warm-up—bicycle—cool down—stretch	4 p.m.	bicycle and shorts	listen to music
Thursday	walk to and from school	morning & afternoon	none	rent a video
Friday	stretch—warm-up—jog 25 minutes—cool down—stretch	after school	jogging shoes, shorts and shirt	proud feeling of accomplishment
Saturday	Basketball	afternoon	tennis shoes and shorts	hang out with friends

Fitness Record

Name _____   Date _____   Period _____

Week of: _____

Day	Activity	Time	Equipment	Reward
Sunday				
Monday				
Tuesday				
Wednesday				
Thursday				
Friday				
Saturday				